CONTENTS

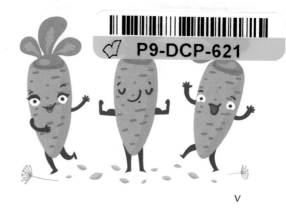

Introduction   v

PART I:
HEALTHY NUTRITION AND
HOMEMADE BABY FOOD   1

Chapter 1:   Why Homemade Baby Food?   3

Chapter 2:   Starting Solids: When, What and How   6

Chapter 3:   Becoming a Baby Food Chef: What You Should
and Shouldn't Feed Your Baby   16

Chapter 4:   The Building Blocks of Good Nutrition   27

Chapter 5:   Safely Feeding Your Baby   39

Chapter 6:   Making Homemade Baby Food 101   45

PART II:
THE RECIPES   61

■ **First Spoonfuls: 6 Months**   63

Vegetable Purees   67

Fruit Purees   75

No-Cook Purees   79

Cereals   83

Tasty Combinations   89

Fun Flavors: 6–8 Months   91

Vibrant Vegetables   95

Fantastic Fruits   101

Mighty Meat and Fish   111

Lovely Legumes   119

More Tasty Combinations   125

Roasted Recipes   135

Tasty Textures: 8–12 Months   139

Great Grains   143

Combination Meals   149

Finger Foods   171

Big Kid Meals: 12 Months and Up   179

Breakfast   185

Lunch and Snacks   197

Soups   221

Dinner   225

Sweet Treats   259

APPENDIX: HEALTH AND NUTRITION RESOURCES   267

INDEX   269

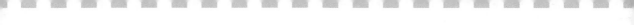

OVER 150 WHOLESOME, NUTRITIOUS RECIPES
FOR YOUR BABY AND TODDLER

natural
BABY FOOD

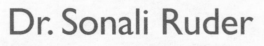

Dr. Sonali Ruder

Creator of the popular food blog *The Foodie Physician*

Hatherleigh Press is committed to preserving and protecting the natural resources of the earth. Environmentally responsible and sustainable practices are embraced within the company's mission statement.

Visit us at www.hatherleighpress.com and register online for free offers, discounts, special events, and more.

Natural Baby Food

Library of Congress Cataloging-in-Publication Data is available upon request.
ISBN: 978-1-57826-604-3

Cover and Interior Design by Carolyn Kasper
Food photography by Peter Fontana
Back cover photo by Luke Fontana

Printed in the United States
10 9 8 7 6 5 4 3 2

INTRODUCTION

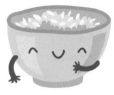

STARTING SOLID FOODS IS one of the biggest milestones in your baby's first year of life. It's also an exciting time for new parents. You and your baby are about to set off on quite an adventure, as you introduce them to a whole new world of flavors. This journey is going to be fun (and messy!), but above all, it will be a significant bonding experience and a learning process for *both* of you.

For some parents, introducing solid foods can be confusing and intimidating. Even though you might be eager to get your baby off to a good culinary start, you may be unsure of how to begin. Most parents have a lot of questions. When should my baby start solids? What should they be eating? What should they avoid? How often should they be eating? How do I know if they've had enough?

I had a lot of the same questions myself when I was a new mom. There are a lot of myths and inconsistencies when it comes to what you should and should not feed your baby, so you may hear conflicting information. Some of this stems from the fact that recommendations have changed a lot in recent years, as more and more research has emerged. Many of the foods that were once forbidden to babies before the one year mark are now allowed, starting at 6 months.

So why homemade baby food? After my daughter Sienna was born, I started making my own baby food because it felt natural for me. After all, I went to culinary school; I cook most of the meals in our household. Making meals for my daughter just felt like an extension of what I was already doing. I'm a foodie after all; I love food, and I wanted to instill that same passion in my daughter.

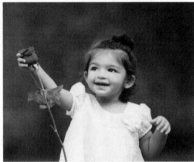

Sonali's daughter, Sienna

But it became so much more than that. I began to realize how important it was for me to start establishing my daughter's healthy eating habits at an early age. The more research I did, the more I realized that dietary patterns are set early in life. Childhood obesity is an epidemic in this country, with 10 percent of children 2–5 years old suffering from obesity. This puts them at a higher risk for chronic conditions like diabetes, high blood pressure, and heart disease. It's crucial to lay the foundation of healthy eating habits from the beginning. Once you start your baby on solids, you have a short but critical window of opportunity to help train their taste buds. By making your own baby food at home, you can use fresh, natural, wholesome ingredients, and teach your baby to appreciate and love the *real* flavors of food.

I wanted to create a comprehensive resource for new parents so that they could get the most pertinent medical and nutritional information, as well as a wide variety of nutritious recipes that would be useful for years to come. Drawing on my background as both a board-certified emergency medicine physician and a chef, this book combines the science of nutrition with the art of cooking to give you the confidence and tools you need to become your baby's own personal chef. Mealtime doesn't have to be stressful or intimidating, and you don't need to be a highly skilled cook to make your own baby food. The truth is, it's actually quite easy.

The recipes in this book are simple and easily adaptable. You can use these recipes from the time your little one takes his or her first bite of solid food, all the way through the toddler years and beyond. The book starts with single ingredient purees for when you first start your baby on solids, and then progresses to combination dishes, incorporating a wide range of flavors and textures. Many of the recipes have optional add-ins like herbs, spices, and other ingredients for a boost of flavor. After all, baby food doesn't have to be bland! Herbs and spices are a great way to add flavor to your baby's food, and many of them also have important health benefits. So start developing your little foodie's palate now!

As children grow up and begin eating from the family table, their diets start to mirror the eating patterns they see in adults and older children. It's for this reason that the last chapter of this book focuses on recipes that are meant to be shared by the whole family. Sitting together at the dinner table and sharing meals is an invaluable experience. You are the best teachers and examples your baby has to follow.

And as soon as your baby is old enough, try to get them in the kitchen with you! I couldn't wait to get Sienna in the kitchen with me. When she was younger, she would sit in her high chair and watch me cook. Now that she's a little older, she's an active participant in the kitchen—mommy's little helper. My heart swells with pride when she asks if she can cook with mommy. Plus, I know that if she helps make a dish, there's a much better chance that she'll eat it. As she grows up, I look forward to spending many hours in the kitchen with her: cooking together, sharing my passion for food, and helping to lay the foundation for a lifetime of healthy eating habits.

My goal is to provide you with the proper information and the confidence to go into the kitchen and do the same with your baby. By reading this book, you've already taken a step in the right direction. By offering your baby a wide variety of healthful and delicious homemade food, you can help them become a well rounded and adventurous eater.

The upcoming months are going to be an exciting time for you and your little one. We've all seen those adorable pictures of babies with food smeared all over their faces. Now it's your turn. These are memories that will last a lifetime, so relax, have fun, and get your camera ready!

Peach Puree,
page 102

Apple Strawberry
Compote, page 130

PART I

HEALTHY NUTRITION AND HOMEMADE BABY FOOD

Goldfish Crackers,
page 203

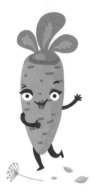

CHAPTER I

Why Homemade Baby Food?

STARTING A BABY ON solid food is not only an exciting time for parents—it's a huge milestone in your baby's life. Over the next several months, you will have almost complete control over your baby's diet, their eating habits, and their developing tastes. By choosing to make your own baby food, you are helping your little one develop a liking for nutritious food from an early age, all while putting them on the path to lifelong healthy eating practices.

As a busy mom, I know that store-bought baby food can sometimes be a necessity, and fortunately there are healthy options available for those hectic times. That being said, nothing beats homemade food. Here are a just a few reasons why:

You are developing your baby's palate for real, natural foods and making them an adventurous eater.
You have a small but critical window of opportunity to develop your baby's palate. In today's world, children are dangerously accustomed to eating processed food: a good percentage of the food that's sold in grocery stores is so artificially colored, sweetened or otherwise enhanced that it's no wonder many children have lost a taste for real food. By making your own baby food at home, you can use fresh, wholesome, natural ingredients while teaching your baby to love the real flavors of food. Babies can also be familiarized with eating the same foods as the rest of the family (just in pureed form), which will make the transition to family meals easier as they get older. In short, exposing your baby to a wide variety of healthful and tasty foods at an early age will help shape their tastes and make him or her a more well-rounded and adventurous eater.

It tastes better and there's more variety.
Commercially prepared baby food can often be bland in taste, aroma, color, and texture. Baby food does not have to be bland! When you make your own baby food, you can use fresh ingredients, which will naturally taste better. Do a taste test and see for yourself: take a bite of jarred baby food and bite of freshly prepared food. Which one looks and smells better? Which one has a fresher taste? Which one would you rather eat?

When you make your own baby food, you can also make use of more diverse ingredients—just try finding avocado or melon in the prepared baby food section. You can try mixing and matching a wide variety of ingredients to create delicious and interesting flavor and texture combinations, rather than being limited by the options at the store. When your baby is ready, you can combine fruits, vegetables, legumes (like lentils and beans), meat, tofu, and the like, to expand their palate and nutritional options. You can also expose them to the world of herbs and spices, which add great flavor to baby food. And by exposing your baby to a wide variety of foods now, he or she will be more likely to try new foods as they get older and grow into the notoriously "picky" toddler age. Children that are consistently fed bland foods are more likely to become picky eaters as they get older, and less likely to try new foods and flavors.

You know exactly what's in your baby's food—and you know it's more nutritious.
Fresh, homemade baby food is more nutritious even at the most basic level. Commercial baby food is heated to very high temperatures in order to sterilize it, so that it can sit on a shelf for long periods of time. This process can kill many important vitamins and minerals, as well as alter the flavor, texture, and aroma of the food. When you make homemade baby food, you can choose cooking methods like steaming and roasting, which help retain these crucial nutrients while maximizing flavor.

Many fruit purees don't even need to be cooked at all, if you use ripe fruit. And that's the benefit of homemade baby food—you can control the ingredients. You *can* use fresh, seasonal fruits and vegetables; you *can* choose to buy organic, or use frozen fruits and vegetables, which are harvested at their nutritional peak. With homemade food, you know exactly what your baby's eating, because you made it. There are no additives like preservatives, starches, and thickeners. While the quality of commercial baby food *has* improved a lot over the years, it may still contain additives, fillers, and empty calories that have no nutritional value.

It's economical and convenient.
Simply put, buying commercial baby food can be expensive. Making food at home, on the other hand, can be very economical. And, believe it or not, it can be just as convenient as store-bought food—if you plan ahead. The keys are in making large batches of baby food and in taking advantage of buying produce in season when prices are lower or buying frozen

fruits and vegetables when they are not in season. These simple tricks result in a diet for your baby that is not only economical but also nutrient-rich. Two large sweet potatoes may cost you about $1.50 at the store, but will make about ten 2-ounce servings of baby food! Compare that to the price of buying the same amount of commercially prepared baby food, and you're definitely coming out ahead.

Some people may find the thought of making homemade food intimidating and time-consuming. The fact is, if you can set aside just one morning or afternoon, you can make enough baby food to last for several weeks. When you prepare large batches of baby food, you can freeze it in individual servings and defrost it as needed. This will help avoid last-minute runs to the grocery store to buy prepared baby food. Most baby food can be stored in the freezer for up to 3 months.

It's fun!

Chances are, once you start making your own baby food at home you're going to find yourself enjoying it—maybe even more than you expected. And, once your baby has a few purees under her or his belt, you can have fun mixing and matching ingredients, coming up with interesting flavor combinations. Let your inner chef really run wild! There's also the inevitable pride factor. There's nothing better than seeing your baby enjoy one of your homemade creations. My daughter tasted a lot of dishes when I was testing recipes for this book and I still love it every time she enthusiastically gobbles up something that I made for her.

To sum it up, making baby food at home is beneficial for both you *and* your baby, for a number of reasons. All you need are some basic tools and few hours in the kitchen. In no time at all, you'll be on your way to becoming a baby food chef. Just by reading this book, you've already taken the first step.

Now, let's get started!

CHAPTER 2

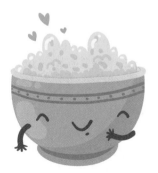

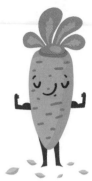

Starting Solids: When, What and How

When Should My Baby Start Solids?

Ideally, most babies should be started on solids around 6 months of age, when they are developmentally ready. The AAP (American Academy of Pediatrics), WHO (World Health Organization) and IOM (Institute of Medicine) all recommend that babies be exclusively breast-fed for the first 6 months of life because of the numerous health benefits of breast-feeding. At about 6 months, they recommend gradually introducing solids, while continuing to breast-feed until the baby's first birthday or longer, if desired. Although experts believe breast milk is the best nutritional choice for infants, in reality, breast-feeding may not be possible for all women. For mothers who are unable to breast-feed (or who decide not to), infant formula is a healthy alternative.

This recommendation stems from the fact that most babies are born with enough iron stores to meet their nutritional needs for approximately their first 6 months of life. After that, your baby's natural iron stores will be depleted, and they will need to get iron from solid foods (in addition to breast milk or formula).

However, every baby develops at a different pace; you may feel that your baby is ready for solids earlier than 6 months. Each child's readiness depends on their own rate of development, so don't rely solely on the calendar! Go by whether your baby is ready—babies must be physically and developmentally ready before they can start on solid foods. Bear in mind that the AAP says it is acceptable to start solids between 4 and 6 months, depending on the individual baby's development. Babies should never start before 4 months. Before 4 months of age, your baby's GI tract is not developed enough to handle digesting solid foods. At this young age, babies still have the extrusion (tongue thrust) reflex, which causes them to push out with their tongues when anything other than liquid is placed in their mouths. Introducing solids too early may also increase your baby's risk of obesity, food allergies, and atopic dermatitis (eczema). Before you start your baby on solid foods, talk to your pediatrician.

Complement, Don't Replace

Calorie for calorie, no solid food has the nutritional quality that breast milk or formula has for your young baby. Breast milk supplies optimal nutrients, antibodies, and other substances that are beneficial for your baby's health. If you feed your baby solid foods too early, their milk intake may decrease, which can interfere with their ability to take in an adequate number of calories or nutrients. You would essentially be replacing milk, the best food for your baby, with foods that are nutritionally inferior and not as easily digested. In fact, solid foods should not be seen as replacements for breast milk; rather, they should complement it. Breast milk or formula will still be the mainstay of your baby's diet for their first year.

An important note: When first starting your baby on solid foods, you are not trying to fill them up. Rather, you are getting them used to the process of eating solids. You're helping your baby learn how to eat, chew, and swallow food. You're introducing them to new tastes and textures. Don't worry if it seems like your baby is more interested in playing with their food rather than eating it; as long as you continue breast milk or formula feedings, you can rest assured that your baby is getting the proper nutrition. Slowly, over the course of the next year, you will wean your baby by gradually reducing the breast milk or formula feedings and increasing the solids.

How Do I Know If My Baby Is Ready?

The best way of knowing when your baby is developmentally ready to start solids is by following their cues.

Here are some signs that your baby may be ready for solids:

- ❀ They can hold their head up on their own. They should be able to sit in a high chair and hold their head up unassisted.
- ❀ They show interest in *your* food. They may open their mouths or lean forward when food comes their way, and seem eager to be fed.
- ❀ They can move food from a spoon to the back of their mouth (i.e. they can swallow food instead of pushing it back out).
- ❀ They have doubled their birth weight

Solids for Better Sleep?

A common reason why parents start their baby on solid foods is because they think it will help their baby sleep through the night. However, the research does not back this up: frequently waking up in the night could be a sign of any number of things besides hunger, such as teething, illness, or a growth spurt. Babies will sleep through the night when they are developmentally mature enough to do so, and are capable of consoling themselves.

How to Get Started

Learning to eat solid food from a spoon is an important developmental milestone in your baby's life. You are opening up a whole new world of flavors for your little one. It's a big transition for your baby, and an important step on their road to independence. You are embarking on an exciting new adventure together!

This will be a significant bonding experience for you and your little one. It will also likely try your patience at times. Don't be surprised if half of the food ends up on the floor during feedings, especially in the beginning! Remember, this is a learning process—for *both* of you. Above all, have fun and try to take it all in stride.

Some tips for feeding your baby solids:

- ❀ Relax. It's normal to be nervous about this milestone. This is a new experience for you and your little one, and it's going to take time to get into a routine. Smile and talk to your baby during feedings. Show the baby how much *you* love the food. Make it playful; your baby will pick up on your cues and it will make the whole experience more pleasant (talking like this also helps with language development).
- ❀ Set aside plenty of time with no distractions. When you first start solids, feedings may take a while. Don't do it when you're in a rush or you'll just get frustrated. Turn off the TV and put away your cell phone. Above all, you want your baby to think of mealtime as a pleasant, relaxing experience.
- ❀ Try introducing solids when your baby is hungry, but *not* starving—you don't want them to be overly cranky. The best time for introducing new solids is a little while after a breast milk or formula feeding. Introducing solids early in the day is preferable, as it lets you watch for any adverse reactions that may occur.
- ❀ Seat your baby upright in a high chair with a supported back, facing forward. Sit directly in front of her or him. It's going to get messy, so coming prepared with a bib and a splash mat on the floor will make cleanup easier.

❀ Use a small, soft-tipped spoon with a long handle, and put just a little bit of food on the tip of the spoon. You can use your finger (pre-washed, of course) as a spoon at first to get your baby used to the idea of eating solids.

❀ Let your baby set the pace for feeding, be it fast or slow. Wait for your baby's cues that she or he wants more before pushing the spoon into his or her mouth. Wait until she or he leans forward and opens his or her mouth, indicating readiness for the next bite. Let the baby continue eating for as long as she or he wants, and knows when to stop. Never force your baby to finish all of the food on the plate. By being responsive to babies in this manner, we are teaching them to listen to their bodies and follow their own cues of hunger and fullness. This ability to self-regulate is a skill that will serve them well throughout life.

Signs That Your Baby Is Full

You'll soon learn to read your baby's signals that they've had enough. Here are a few common signs:

- ♥ Turns head away
- ♥ Leans back in the chair
- ♥ Closes or purses lips
- ♥ Spits out the food
- ♥ Plays with the food
- ♥ Tries to knock the spoon out of your hand

Can I Put Solids in My Baby's Bottle?

Putting cereals or other solids in your baby's bottle is not a good idea, for a few reasons. In addition to being a choking hazard, it can cause delays in your baby learning important feeding skills. It may also cause your baby to overeat. When you feed your baby from a spoon, they are able to rest between bites and get a sense for when they feel full. Babies learn to self-regulate this way. Also, giving solids in a bottle may lead to your replacing breast milk or formula, which is packed with essential nutrients that your baby needs. To sum it up, always use a spoon.

Follow the 3–5 Day Rule

Introduce solid foods one at a time, for 3–5 days; that way, if your baby has an adverse reaction, you'll be more likely to know which food caused it. You can also note which foods they seem to prefer and which ones they don't. If your baby makes faces when you offer them a certain food, that doesn't necessarily mean they don't like it. It could just be that it's new and different, and they need time to get used to it. Be persistent, and offer it again at another time. Research indicates that some babies need multiple exposures to a new taste before they learn to enjoy it. In fact, it can take as many as *10–15 tries* before a baby accepts a new food!

Once your baby begins tolerating a few single ingredients, you can start giving food in combinations. This is when you can let your creative side shine, and the fun really begins! Have fun experimenting, and don't let your own preconceptions about what tastes good affect what you feed your baby. *You* may not be a fan of beets, but don't let that stop you from feeding them to your baby! (In fact, babies often enjoy beets because of their sweet flavor and bright color.) Have fun mixing and matching; while you may not necessarily think to combine fruits and vegetables like broccoli, peas, and pears, it might just be a combination that your baby loves!

One last note: don't expect your baby to eat the same amount at every meal. An infant's appetite varies from meal to meal. Sometimes, you'll be shocked at how much your little guy or girl is eating; other times, you'll be frustrated that your baby isn't interested in the food at all. This is all completely normal!

Which Solids Should I Introduce First?

The rules about when to introduce certain foods to your baby's diet have changed a lot in recent years. Pediatricians used to recommend delaying the introduction of highly allergenic foods like egg whites, fish, and peanuts, but the AAP now gives these foods the green light at 6 months. (You can read more about this in Chapter 5: Safely Feeding Your Baby.)

While iron-fortified white rice cereal is the most commonly recommended first food by pediatricians, this is based more on tradition than science. Rice cereal is easily digestible and non-allergenic, which is why it's traditionally been recommended. But the truth is, other than its being fortified with iron, rice cereal is actually not a very nutritious first food—it's a refined grain and is low in protein. The AAP now states that *there's no medical evidence that introducing solid foods in any particular order has an advantage for your baby*. In fact, you may just as well start with a vegetable or fruit puree. Meats can also be introduced at an early age. Meats are good sources of high-quality protein and are rich in iron and zinc, which are crucial for your developing baby. The current recommendations are that meats, such as turkey, chicken, and beef should be one of the first solids added to a breast-fed infant's diet, because breast milk is typically low in these nutrients. Beans and legumes like chickpeas and lentils are great vegetarian sources of protein, and are also high in iron. If you *are* going to start with a cereal, there are plenty of nutritious whole grain options, like brown rice cereal, barley, or oatmeal.

Vegetables before Fruits?

You may have heard people say that you should start with a vegetable rather than a fruit puree, so that your baby does not develop a sweet tooth. However, there is no research to support this claim; in fact, amniotic fluid and breast milk are both sweet in their own right, so babies may already have a predilection for sweet foods from birth. The bottom line? Feeding your baby a wide range of nutritious foods is more important than the order in which you introduce them.

How Much and How Often Should I Feed My Baby?

There's no mathematical formula to tell you how much food you should feed your baby. Your pediatrician may give you a sample feeding schedule to give you an idea of how much your baby should be eating, but every baby progresses at a different pace—you will need to follow their lead. Start with solids once a day while continuing to breast-feed or give formula. Increase to two solid meals a day and gradually work your way up until you're giving your baby solids three times a day. Note that this can take a couple of months. By around 8–9 months, most babies will be eating three solid food meals per day. Also, slowly increase the amount of food you give at each feeding. Start with about 1–2 tablespoons of solids at each feeding and increase it over the next couple of months to ¼ cup, and then ½ cup (4 ounces) or more. Again, there is no exact amount as to how much solid food your baby should be eating, as every baby is different, and the amount they eat will vary a lot from meal to meal.

Throughout this whole process, it is important to continue to give breast milk or formula between or with feedings. After you introduce solids, babies still need about 24–32 ounces of breast milk or formula a day, divided into 4–5 feedings. While solids provide some nutrients and calories, the small amounts your baby will be starting with aren't enough to sustain them. Remember, breast milk or formula is still going to be your baby's primary source of nutrition. The amount of breast milk or formula your baby needs will decrease over time as your baby transitions fully to solids.

Within a few months of starting solid foods, your baby's daily diet should include a wide variety of healthy foods that may include the following:

- Breast milk and/or formula
- Meats
- Cereal
- Vegetables
- Fruits
- Eggs
- Fish

Progressing Through the Stages of Solids

As you introduce your baby to solid foods, the type and texture of the foods you offer will change as they grow. In the beginning, you will want to start with single-ingredient purees, with a very thin, almost watery consistency. As your baby progresses, you will start to thicken your purees more and add more ingredients. Eventually, you will forgo the smooth purees and move on to chunkier purees. Instead of using your blender or food processor, you'll start mashing your ingredients together with a fork or potato masher to get your baby accustomed to new textures. Finally, your baby will move on to table food, which can be chopped into bite-size pieces.

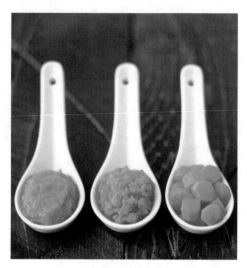

In general, your baby will become accustomed to new textures at the following rate:

- ❀ 4–6 months: runny, thin, smooth
- ❀ 6–8 months: pureed
- ❀ 8–12: pureed and mashed; soft finger foods
- ❀ 12–18 months: mashed and chopped

4–6 Months

When your baby first begins solids, you will begin by giving her or him single ingredient foods. While single-grain cereals like rice, barley, or oatmeal are common first foods, you can just as easily start with a single-vegetable or single-fruit puree. Starchy, sweet vegetables like sweet potatoes, squash, and peas are all good choices. Mild, low-acid fruits like apple and pear also make for nice options. Or, if you prefer, you can start with a simple, no-cook puree like avocado or banana.

No matter what you choose to feed your baby first, the texture should be smooth, thin, and runny when you first start. You can thin the puree as needed with breast milk or formula, so that it maintains a semi-liquid consistency. For the first few feedings, begin with a couple of teaspoons of food. As your baby gets used to the idea of eating from a spoon, the teaspoons will soon turn to tablespoons.

6–8 Months

Continue giving your baby a wide variety of single purees, and start combining them to broaden their palate. You can begin to introduce all sorts of fruits, like peaches, cherries, and melons. Include different-colored vegetables, like green beans, cauliflower, and beets. You can also introduce pureed meat like beef, chicken, turkey, or lamb, which are all good sources of iron, a critical mineral that your baby needs at this age. You can also introduce beans and legumes like black beans, lentils, and split peas, which are high in protein and iron. While you should still hold off on cow's milk until your baby is 1 year's old, you can introduce yogurt, eggs, and some cheese (like cottage cheese and cheddar), which are more easily tolerated.

As you expand your baby's palate, make sure to introduce new ingredients one at a time to watch for any adverse reactions. Make combination purees with ingredients you've already introduced, and be creative. Try my Pretty in Pink Raspberry Pear Puree (page 108) or Gingery Carrots and Apples (page 127). Start using herbs and spices to flavor your baby's food—baby food does not have to be bland!

In addition to introducing your baby to a wide variety of new foods, you should gradually thicken the consistency of your purees as your baby tolerates it. You can do this by using less breast milk or formula to thin your purees, or else by adding a small amount of cereal to thicken it.

During this time, you can start to introduce formula, breast milk, or water in a sippy cup at meals.

8–12 Months

As your baby gets older, they will become better at chewing. You can start making food with a lumpier, mashed consistency, rather than smooth purees. During this period, you'll be using your blender or food processor less, and using a fork or potato masher more. You can start introducing finely minced meat (as tolerated) instead of pureed. Although babies won't develop their molars until about age 1, they are very effective at mashing food between their gums. Continue to expand your baby's palate by offering new meats, beans, legumes, tofu, whole grains, fruits, and vegetables in interesting combinations. Continue to increase the amount of food you give at feedings, following your baby's cues.

Start giving your baby combination meals, which combine fruits, vegetables, proteins, grains, and dairy. Examples would be my Peachy Banana Oatmeal with Yogurt (page 150), Chicken, Mango and Quinoa (page 160) or Salmon with Lentils and Carrots (page 166). Introduce more herbs and spices to expand your baby's palate, such as with Baby's Chicken Curry (page 163)—a good recipe to try and one that the whole family can enjoy.

By 8–10 months, infants begin to develop the pincer grasp, which lets them pick up objects between their thumb and forefinger. At this point, your little one will be ready to start trying finger foods, and may not want purees anymore. As their self-feeding skills improve, they will want to start eating independently, play with their food, and hold their own cup. Introduce finger foods like cooked, soft pieces of carrots or sweet potato, O-shaped cereal, small pieces of ripe pear or peach, small pasta, or scrambled eggs (see page 172 for more finger food ideas).

You can also introduce limited amounts of 100 percent fruit juice in a cup (no more than 4 ounces per day; see The Scoop on Juice on page 26).

12 Months and Up

Your little one has now been introduced to all of the different foods groups, and has quite a bit of experience under her or his belt! If you haven't done so already, pull their chair up to the table so that they can participate in family meals. At this age, they can eat table food that is cut into small pieces, like pasta, stews, and quesadillas. Encourage self-feeding with utensils and start phasing out formula and baby purees. Continue to offer your baby, as well as the rest of the family, a wide variety of textures, tastes, and food experiences.

You can now introduce ingredients like cow's milk and honey. You can also season your child's food with a small amount of salt. Although you don't want to go crazy with the salt shaker, the amount of salt you add to homemade food is invariably less than the amount of salt found in packaged and processed foods.

With age comes increasing independence. Your little one may soon become more interested in walking and exploring than in sitting still and eating. Toddlers' eating habits are notoriously unpredictable, but try to eat together as a family as often as possible. If your little ones see the rest of the family enjoying their food, it will encourage them to eat. Also, it's okay to let them play with their food—eating should be an enjoyable experience, and playing with their food is a totally normal way for babies to learn to accept foods that are new and different.

Around this age, start offering 2–3 nutritious snacks a day in addition to meals. Some examples of healthy snacks are my Zucchini Tots (page 198), Crispy Tofu Nuggets

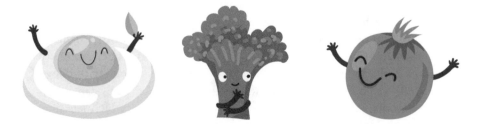

(page 200) and Avocado Egg Salad (page 204). Don't worry if your toddler doesn't eat consistent amounts at every meal. Although this may be frustrating, it is completely normal. Your job is to offer nutritious, tasty food choices at meal and snack times. Your child's job is to choose how much they eat of the foods you serve. Over time, they will get all the nutrients they need to grow.

Stool School

After you start solids, you may notice some big changes going on in your baby's diaper (some not so pleasant)! It's normal for your baby's stool to change in color and odor when you add solids to their diet. Peas and spinach may turn the stool a green color, sweet potatoes and carrots can give it an orange hue, and beets may make it red. If your purees are not completely strained, you may find little pieces of undigested food in the stool, like bits of corn or peas. This is all completely normal, and is a result of your baby's digestive system needing time to mature fully.

If your baby develops constipation, which is common after the introduction of solids, you may want to cut back on foods like rice cereal, applesauce, bananas, and dairy, and instead incorporate foods that can help alleviate constipation like pears, peaches, prunes, and papaya. You can also try barley or oatmeal cereal instead of rice cereal. If your baby has discomfort, gas, or watery, runny stool after eating a specific food, stop giving it for a few weeks and then try again. If the problem continues, consult your pediatrician.

As you begin on this journey of introducing solid foods to your baby, remember that every child develops at a different pace. The rule of thumb is to watch your baby—not the calendar!

CHAPTER 3

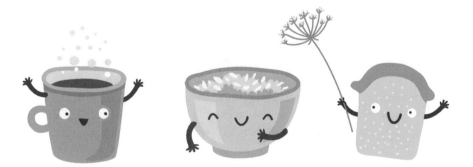

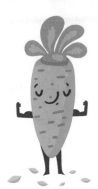

Becoming a Baby Food Chef: What You Should and Shouldn't Feed Your Baby

Healthy cooking for babies and toddlers is really not all that different from healthy cooking for adults. That being said, there are a few things that you need to know, as well as some ingredients that should be limited in your baby's diet. No one is going to have as much influence over your baby's diet in the upcoming months and years as you, so it's important that you know how to offer your baby a balanced diet, filled with a wide range of nutritious, whole foods.

Whole foods are foods that are as close to their natural state as possible. These nutritionally dense foods provide many important vitamins and minerals that nourish your baby and fuel his or her growth and development. Focus on choosing whole foods as much as possible, as opposed to over-processed and refined foods that are filled with empty calories.

One of the best ways to ensure that your baby (and the rest of your family) follows a nutritious diet is to cook at home, where there's no question as to what goes into your food. Cooking at home is healthier than eating out or buying packaged food from the grocery store; when you cook at home, you can choose the best quality ingredients and use healthy cooking techniques to maximize the flavor and nutrients in your baby's food.

Cooking at home will also help to set a good example for your baby, instilling healthy eating habits at an early age. Once they are old enough to join you in the kitchen, teaching your children to cook is a gift of health and independence that they will use for their entire lives.

What You *Should* Feed Your Baby

Do give your baby a wide range of nutrient-dense whole foods, including:

- ❀ Vegetables
- ❀ Fruits
- ❀ Whole grains

- ❀ Meat, poultry and eggs
- ❀ Seafood

- ❀ Dairy
- ❀ Beans and other legumes

Sweet Potato and
Kale Quesadillas
page 247

HEALTHY FOODS FOR BABY

Vegetables and Fruits	Offer a rainbow of colorful vegetables and fruits; they are packed with important vitamins like vitamin A and C, as well as minerals like folate. They are also rich in phytonutrients, plant-based compounds that are beneficial for your baby's health.
Whole Grains	Whole grains like brown rice, barley, oatmeal, whole wheat pasta, whole wheat bread, whole wheat crackers and teething biscuits are packed with complex carbohydrates. At least half of all grains that your baby eats should be whole grains. Iron-fortified cereals can help your baby get the iron they need. Be cautious with high-fiber foods like bran cereal, which is low in calories but high in bulk; while these foods are good for adults, in babies they can fill their stomachs quickly, leaving less room for other nutrients.
Meat, Poultry and Eggs	Offer a variety of soft, pureed or finely chopped meats like chicken, turkey, beef, lamb or pork, as well as eggs. These are all valuable sources of protein, which is needed for growth. Iron and zinc, which are higher in red meat like beef and lamb (and dark-meat chicken and turkey), are crucial for your baby's cognitive development, growth and immune system.
Seafood	An important source of lean protein, as well as the omega-3 fatty acids DHA and EPA. They are crucial for the development of your baby's brain and eyes. Make sure to always choose low mercury seafood.
Dairy	A primary source of calcium for your baby, dairy is also rich in protein. Yogurt, cheese, ricotta cheese and cottage cheese can be given before 12 months; after 12 months, cow's milk is an important source of calories and nutrients. Don't give low-fat or fat-free milk products to children under two years of age unless instructed by your doctor. Always give pasteurized milk products.
Beans and other Legumes	Beans (like black, kidney and pinto), lentils, chickpeas and soybeans are excellent vegetarian sources of protein and are rich in complex carbohydrates; they also are good sources of folate and iron. Unlike meat sources of protein, these are usually incomplete proteins, so eat a wide variety for best results.

Do Use Herbs and Spices to Season Your Baby's Food

Baby food does not need to be bland! If you look at other cultures around the world, including India, the Middle East, and Latin America, people introduce their babies from an early age to a wide variety of food with complex flavors. Don't be afraid of herbs and spices; they are a great way to add flavor (as well as antioxidants) to your baby's food without adding less desirable ingredients like sugar or salt.

Babies palates are actually influenced by the food you eat while they're still in the womb. After they're born, the foods and flavors you eat continue to be transmitted to them through breast milk, so if you're eating highly seasoned food, your baby has already been exposed to a wide variety of flavors. In other words, it's almost a step backward to start feeding your baby bland food when you introduce them to solids.

The eating habits you establish in your baby are going to continue into toddlerhood and beyond, so don't let them get stuck in a bland food rut! Babies who are exposed to a wide variety of flavors at a young age are more likely to be adventurous eaters as they grow up.

In addition to expanding your baby's palate, many herbs and spices have health benefits. For centuries, herbs and spices have been used for medicinal purposes; many, like basil, cinnamon, oregano, thyme, and rosemary, are packed with antioxidants that help fight chronic diseases like cancer, diabetes, and heart disease. Others like cloves, turmeric, and allspice, help curb inflammation in the body. Some, like garlic, nutmeg, and cumin, also have antimicrobial properties that help fight infection. Still others, like ginger, coriander, and mint, are known to aid in digestion and soothe an upset tummy.

Herbs and spices are traditionally defined as any part of a plant that is used in the diet for their aromatic properties. Although the terms are often used interchangeably, there is a difference between the two. Herbs refer to the leafy portions of a plant and can be fresh or dried. Examples are basil, rosemary, parsley, and thyme. Spices, on the other hand, are harvested from any other portion of the plant and are typically dried. Popular spices come from berries (peppercorns), roots (ginger), seeds (nutmeg), flower buds (cloves), and even the stamens of flowers (saffron). Some plants give both an herb and a spice—cilantro is the leafy herb from the same plant that gives us coriander seed.

Dried herbs are stronger and have a more concentrated flavor than fresh herbs, so if a recipe calls for a fresh herb and you want to use dried, you should make certain to use less. A general rule of thumb is that dried herbs are about three times as strong as fresh herbs, so if you're substituting dried herbs in a recipe, use a third of the amount listed. For example, if a recipe calls for 3 teaspoons of fresh thyme and you only have dried, use 1 teaspoon. Crush dried herbs in your fingers to release their flavors before adding them to a dish. One final note: dried spices can start to lose their flavor if they've been sitting on a shelf for a while, so try toasting whole or ground spices in a skillet to liven up their flavor.

Herbs and spices can be used in both sweet and savory dishes. Some herbs, like bay leaves, rosemary, and thyme, are hearty herbs that should be cooked for a long time with the food. Add them early in the cooking process for dishes like soups and stews where they will slowly infuse their flavor with time. These sturdy herbs can also withstand high temperatures in the oven and work well in dishes like oven-roasted vegetables and chicken. Other herbs, like chives and basil, are more delicate and should be added at the end of the cooking process to add bright, fresh flavor to a dish. Introduce herbs and spices to your baby's diet one at a time, just like any other new ingredient, so that you can watch for adverse reactions. Many of the recipes throughout this book have optional suggestions for herbs, spices, or other ingredients to boost the flavor of the dish. These are designated as "Flavor Boost."

HERBS AND THEIR USES

HERB:	FLAVOR PROFILE:	PAIRS WELL WITH:
Basil	Delicate, sweet, warm, aromatic herb, which is a staple in Southern European cuisine. Thai basil, used in Asian cuisine, has a slight spice and licorice-like flavor.	Strawberries, lemon, peaches
		Carrots, corn, green beans, eggplant, tomatoes, red peppers, potatoes, zucchini
		Beans, chicken, fish, lamb
		Olive oil, pesto, and pasta dishes
Bay leaves	Woodsy, sharp warm flavor; slowly releases flavor, so best used to add depth of flavor to soups and stews that take a while to cook	Apples, figs
		Cauliflower, potatoes, pumpkin, tomatoes
		Fish, poultry, meats
		Rice, dried beans, soups, stock
Chives	Delicate, mild onion flavor; in the same family as onions, leeks, and garlic	Avocados, potatoes, parsnips
		Chicken, eggs, fish
		Sauces, salads, and soups
Cilantro	Complex, pungent, herbaceous flavor; one of the most commonly used herbs in the world, especially in Caribbean, Latin American, and Asian cooking	Avocados, mango, citrus
		Bell peppers, carrots, corn, potatoes, tomatoes
		Chicken, meats, seafood, yogurt
		Dried beans, lentils, coconut milk, rice, curries, salsa
Dill weed	Delicate, feathery leaves; pungent herb flavor	Beets, cabbage, carrots, cucumber, green beans, peas, potatoes, tomatoes
		Eggs, salmon, yogurt
		Sauces

HERBS AND THEIR USES

HERB:	FLAVOR PROFILE:	PAIRS WELL WITH:
Mint	Fresh, cool, intense, aromatic; used in sweet and savory dishes	Berries, mango, melon, papaya, pineapple
		Asparagus, carrots, cucumber, eggplant, green beans, peas, zucchini
		Fish, lamb, yogurt
Marjoram	Floral and woodsy; similar to oregano but milder	Asparagus, green beans, mushrooms, potatoes, spinach, summer squash, tomatoes, zucchini
		Chicken, fish, meats
		Pasta
Oregano	Robust, strong, earthy flavor; common in Italian, Mexican, and Mediterranean cuisine	Bell peppers, broccoli, mushrooms, potatoes, summer squash, tomatoes, zucchini
		Beef, fish, poultry, pork,
		Dried beans, pasta, and pasta sauces
Parsley	Bright, grassy, light; comes in flat leaf (Italian) or curly varieties	Avocado, broccoli, carrots, parsnips, potatoes, tomatoes, zucchini
		Chicken, fish, meats
		Grains, salads, stews, stock, pasta, and pasta sauces
Rosemary	Bold and piney flavor	Pears
		Butternut squash, potatoes, pumpkin
		Beef, chicken, lamb
		Lentils, dried beans, soups, stews
Sage	Warm, earthy flavor	Butternut squash, parsnips, pumpkin
		Poultry, pork, sausage
		Dried beans, stuffing
Tarragon	Anise, licorice-like flavor; common in French cuisine	Asparagus, broccoli, carrots, cauliflower, potatoes, tomatoes
		Chicken, lamb, seafood
		Sauces
Thyme	Robust, woodsy	Blueberries
		Beets, butternut squash, carrots, mushrooms, parsnips, potatoes, zucchini
		Beef, fish, lamb, poultry, pork
		Soups, stews, stock, lentils, dried beans

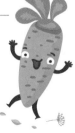

SPICES AND THEIR USES

SPICE:	FLAVOR PROFILE:	PAIRS WELL WITH:
Allspice	Warm, sweet, and intense flavor reminiscent of cloves, cinnamon, and nutmeg; popular in Caribbean cuisine	Apples, pears, pineapple, plums Beets, pumpkin, squash, sweet potatoes Beef, chicken Stewed dishes, baked goods
Cardamom	Warm, aromatic, spicy, sweet flavor with floral hints; common in Indian cuisine	Apples, apricots, bananas, dates, oranges Carrots, winter squash Chicken, lamb, yogurt Curries, rice dishes, desserts
Chili powder (blend)	Blend of spices like cayenne pepper, cumin, oregano, garlic; used in Mexican and Southwest cuisine	Avocado, corn, tomatoes Meats, poultry, Dried beans, lentils, chili, stews, rice, sauces
Cinnamon	Sweet and lightly spicy flavor with an intense fragrance; there are hundreds of types of cinnamon, but the most common one is Ceylon; can be used in sweet or savory dishes	Apples, bananas, blueberries, cherries, pears, plums Carrots, eggplant, pumpkin, sweet potatoes, winter squash Chicken, meats, pork, ricotta cheese Nuts, oatmeal, rice, desserts
Cloves	Strong, sweet, fruity taste that's also pungent and leaves a lingering flavor; can overpower other seasonings, so use sparingly	Apples, orange, plums Pumpkin, sweet potatoes, tomatoes Ham, chicken, beef, lamb Baked goods, stews
Coriander	Bright, earthy, lemony; from the same plant as cilantro	Orange, pears, plums Carrots, potatoes, spinach Chicken, seafood, pork Lentils, chickpeas, curries
Cumin	Earthy, smoky; common in Southwest, Mexican, North African, Middle Eastern, and Indian cuisine	Carrots, eggplant, squash, sweet potatoes, tomatoes Beef, chicken, lamb, pork Dried beans, chickpeas, chili, lentils
Curry powder (blend)	Blend of Indian spices; ranges from mild to spicy (start with mild for babies)	Carrots, cauliflower, parsnips, potatoes, tomatoes, zucchini Chicken, meats, seafood Coconut milk, rice

SPICES AND THEIR USES

SPICE:	FLAVOR PROFILE:	PAIRS WELL WITH:
Garlic	Although technically not really an herb or spice, garlic is available fresh or as garlic powder, which is made from dehydrated garlic cloves; aromatic with a mildly spicy flavor; garlic powder has a milder flavor than raw garlic; good in "no-cook" dishes when you don't want a very pungent garlic flavor	Broccoli, eggplant, green beans, potatoes, spinach, tomatoes, zucchini Chicken, meats, seafood Dried beans, lentils, pasta and pasta sauces, soups, stock
Ginger	Fragrant with a slightly sweet, hot flavor; common in Asian cuisine	Apples, mango, pears, peaches, plums Beets, broccoli, butternut squash, carrots, green beans, parsnips, sweet potatoes Meats, poultry Curries, rice
Nutmeg	Warm, slightly sweet and spicy; strong, so use sparingly; used in sweet and savory dishes	Apples, pears, peaches, dried fruit Carrots, parsnips, potatoes, pumpkin, spinach, sweet potatoes Chicken, lamb, ricotta cheese Oatmeal, cream sauces, pasta, rice pudding
Paprika	Slightly sweet and bitter, adds red color to dishes; comes in sweet, smoked and spicy varieties; common in Spanish and Hungarian cuisine	Bell peppers, cauliflower, mushrooms, potatoes Beef, chicken, eggs, fish, lamb, pork Chickpeas, lentils, stews, goulash
Pepper	Pungent with mild heat; comes in variety of colors like black, white, pink, and green; ranges from mild to pungent	Apricots, strawberries, cherries All vegetables Eggs, meats, poultry, seafood
Turmeric	Warm, earthy, mild woodsy flavor; adds yellow color; common in Indian, Thai, and Moroccan cuisine	Cauliflower, eggplant, potatoes, spinach Beef, chicken, eggs, lamb, seafood Curries, rice, lentils, coconut milk, sauces
Vanilla	Strongly aromatic, warm and gentle; vanilla extract often contains alcohol, so check the label or else use whole vanilla beans	Apples, apricots, banana, pears, peaches, plums, strawberries Ricotta cheese, yogurt Oatmeal, baked goods, desserts

What You Should *Not* Feed Your Baby
Don't Give Cow's Milk before 1 Year

Whole cow's milk should be avoided until your baby's first birthday, for a few reasons. First of all, whole milk should never be used to replace breast milk or formula, both of which contain vitamins, minerals, and essential fatty acids that cow's milk just doesn't have. For example, cow's milk has low iron content, and also contains compounds that inhibit your baby's ability to absorb iron. In addition, your baby's immature kidneys can't handle the high levels of protein and minerals in cow's milk. Some babies may also have difficulty digesting the proteins as well as the sugar lactose.

Yogurt and some cheeses can be introduced before your baby is 1 year old (see box below), but as with all new foods, it's important to watch out for any signs of allergy or digestive discomfort when introducing dairy foods to your baby. At 1 year old, babies can be transitioned to full fat cow's milk instead of formula or breast milk. After age 2, babies can be switched from whole milk to reduced-fat milk and dairy products.

Milk vs. Yogurt (and Cheese)

Although cow's milk is not recommended before your baby's first birthday, as mentioned you *can* introduce dairy products like yogurt and cheese earlier. Why? Because the culturing process results in the breakdown of lactose, making yogurt and cheese easier to digest. Greek yogurt in particular is extensively strained, which removes a lot of the lactose content. Hard, aged cheeses, like cheddar and Swiss, have even less lactose. The culturing process also modifies the milk proteins, making these products less allergenic than milk. Giving your baby whole milk yogurt and cheese lets them gain access to the healthy fats they need. These foods are also a good source of protein and calcium. Don't buy pre-sweetened yogurts; stir in a little fresh fruit puree instead.

Don't Give Honey before 1 Year

Honey can be contaminated by botulism spores, which produce toxins that can be harmful to your baby. Adults and babies over 1 year are able to fight off these toxins; however, young babies don't have the immune system to cope with the toxins.

Don't Give Sugar before 1 Year

You should avoid using sugar and other sweeteners in your baby's food before their first birthday. You want your baby to appreciate the natural taste of food; children today consume far too much sugar. Sugar contains empty calories that fill your baby up, leaving less room for nutritious foods. If you want to add sweetness to a dish, add some fruit puree.

Don't Give Salt before 1 Year

Babies don't require much sodium, and too much salt can actually strain your baby's kidneys. Instead of salt, use herbs and spices to season your baby's food. After 1 year, you can use a small amount of salt to season their food. Contrary to what you may think, the salt shaker is not the main cause of too much sodium in the diet. Rather, most of our dietary sodium intake comes from eating packaged and restaurant foods. Learn to read the labels on packaged food before giving them to your little one. Foods like jarred tomato sauce, canned soup, and packaged macaroni and cheese are often loaded with sodium.

Don't Give Small, Round Foods That Are Choking Hazards

Foods like whole nuts, hot dog pieces, popcorn, whole grapes, chunks of meat or cheese, and raw vegetables are choking hazards and should be avoided. Also, don't give your baby sticky foods like marshmallows or chewing gum. Nut butters like peanut or almond butter are okay, but should be spread thinly on bread or crackers, not given in large spoonfuls or chunks.

Don't Give Raw Milk Cheeses

Pasteurization is a process that kills bacteria through heating. Some cheeses, especially soft cheeses like Brie, feta, Camembert, Roquefort, and Mexican cheeses like queso blanco and queso fresco, are more likely to contain unpasteurized milk and should be avoided. Firm cheeses like cheddar and Swiss are generally safe, but remember to read labels and make sure the products are made with pasteurized milk.

Don't Give Undercooked or Raw Meat, Seafood, or Eggs

Cook meat, poultry, fish, and eggs fully to kill any potentially harmful bacteria. Refer to the Food Temperature Guide (page 55) to see the safe minimum internal temperatures for these foods.

Don't Give Low-Fat Foods before 2 Years

Children under two years old need to get a high percentage of their calories from fat in order to promote proper growth, and in order for brain development to occur at the proper rate. Full fat products, like whole milk and whole milk yogurt and cheese, should be given to your baby unless your pediatrician specifies otherwise (they may recommend low-fat products if your baby is at risk for obesity or heart disease). After your baby's second birthday, you can switch to reduced-fat milk and dairy products.

The Scoop on Juice

Hold off on giving juice to your baby to give them a chance to develop a taste for water. Juice is not a nutrient-dense food; it doesn't have the fiber and other nutrients found in whole fruits and vegetables, and it can be high in sugar. It's also less filling than breast milk or formula, so infants can consume a lot of it without feeling full and thus can overdrink it. Drinking too much juice can also cause diarrhea, and can contribute to poor nutrition, obesity, and tooth decay.

When you *do* give your child juice, make sure it is 100 percent, unsweetened juice. A good option is to dilute juice with water before introducing it to your baby. In fact, the AAP recommends waiting until a baby is at least 6–9 months of age before giving them juice, and then only in limited amounts. Encourage whole fruits instead. For children ages 1–6 years old, limit fruit juice consumption to 4–6 ounces (½–¾ cup) per day. Any more than this will reduce their appetite for other, more nutritious foods.

Offer juice only with a meal or snack, rather than letting your child sip it throughout the day or at bedtime. Always offer it in a cup rather than a bottle.

Cooking for your baby is easy, as long as you follow a few basic guidelines. As your baby's palate expands, you can have fun experimenting with new flavors, provided you know which ingredients you should limit. By preparing nutritious, wholesome and tasty food for your little one, you are developing healthy eating habits early and giving them the best possible start in life.

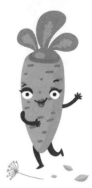

CHAPTER 4

The Building Blocks of Good Nutrition

G OOD NUTRITION IS ESSENTIAL for the substantial growth and development that occurs during your baby's first year of life. Did you know that during infancy, the nutrient requirements per pound of body weight are proportionally higher than at any other time in our lives? In order for these crucial changes to occur properly, your baby must obtain an adequate amount of essential nutrients. During the first several months, when you were solely breast-feeding or bottle feeding, you didn't really need to think about your baby's nutrition too much—things were on autopilot. But once you introduce solids into your baby's diet, it becomes important to learn how best to provide your little one with a balanced, nutritious diet.

While it's true that during the first year of your baby's life, breast milk or formula will continue to be your baby's primary source of nutrition, as you begin to phase out breast milk and increase solids, your baby is going to have to start getting their essential nutrients from eating the right types and amounts of solid food. By feeding your baby a well-balanced diet, full of the main nutritional building blocks, you start them on the path to lifelong good health.

Five Main Nutritional Building Blocks

Simply put, nutrients are the substances needed for growth, metabolism, and other body functions. They are divided into *macronutrients* (which include carbohydrates, protein and fat) and *micronutrients* (which include vitamins and minerals).

The five main building blocks of nutrition are:

- Proteins
- Carbohydrates
- Fats
- Vitamins
- Minerals

Macronutrients
Powerful Proteins

Protein is the structural component of every part of your baby's body. Proteins are responsible for building, maintaining, and repairing new tissue, so it is crucial for your baby's diet to include enough protein to fuel this period of rapid growth and development.

Proteins are made up of smaller building blocks called amino acids. Animal sources of protein, like beef, chicken, fish, and dairy products, tend to be *complete* proteins, which means they contain all of the amino acids that are required by your body. Plant-based protein sources, like beans, seeds, vegetables, grains, and nuts are usually *incomplete* proteins, meaning that they lack one or more of the amino acids that your body can't produce. There are a few vegetarian foods like soy, quinoa, and chia seeds that are complete proteins.

Giving your baby a wide variety of protein sources is the best way to ensure that they are getting all of their essential amino acids. The key is in combining complementary proteins to make complete proteins. By combining legumes with grains, or grains with dairy, for example, you can completely satisfy your baby's amino acid needs. And there's no need to worry about giving your baby protein sources together in a single meal—as long as your baby gets them throughout the day, his or her needs will be fulfilled.

Here are a few nutritious examples of complementary protein combinations:

- Brown rice and beans
- Peanut or almond butter on whole wheat bread
- Whole grain cereal or oatmeal with milk
- Pasta with cheese or meat sauce
- Quesadilla with pinto beans spread on a whole wheat tortilla
- Split pea soup with barley
- Yogurt with wheat germ
- Hummus with whole wheat crackers

Good Protein Sources for Baby and Toddler

- ♥ Meat and poultry: chicken, turkey, beef, lamb, pork
- ♥ Seafood: salmon, cod, haddock, etc.
- ♥ Eggs
- ♥ Dairy: yogurt (especially Greek yogurt), cheese, cottage cheese, milk (after 1 year)
- ♥ Legumes: tofu, soybeans, dried beans, dried peas, lentils, chickpeas
- ♥ Nuts and seeds (ground or made into butter, not given whole): peanut butter, almond butter, sunflower seed butter, sesame seed paste (tahini)
- ♥ Whole grains: wheat, oats, barley, quinoa, rice, millet, amaranth, corn
- ♥ Fruits and vegetables: avocado, dried fruit (apricots, prunes, dates, raisins), peas, green beans, potatoes, broccoli, kale

---

Crucial Carbohydrates

Carbohydrates are your baby's main source of fuel. They are broken down into glucose, which the body can use immediately to provide energy, or else they can be stored for later use. Many cells in our bodies (like brain cells) must have glucose to stay alive, which is why it's so important to get enough carbohydrates. If you don't eat enough carbohydrates, your body will start to break down vital proteins for energy.

With all of the bad nutritional press that sugars get, it can be very confusing for new parents to decide what to feed their babies and toddlers. The key is choosing the *right* sugars. *Simple carbohydrates* or sugars are small molecules of sugar that are easily processed by the body and provide a quick energy boost. They are found in foods like table sugar, high fructose corn syrup, cakes, cookies, candy, and sweetened beverages. These types of sugars provide calories, but with few nutrients. Because the body breaks them down quickly, they also give you a quick energy boost, but then leave you feeling cranky and tired later. You should limit the amount of simple sugars in your child's diet. In fact, you shouldn't be adding any sugar or sweetener to your baby's food at all during the first year; rather, let them learn to appreciate the natural taste of food.

Choose *complex carbohydrates* instead. Because it takes your body longer to process complex carbohydrates, they are more satisfying and provide long-lasting energy for your little one. They also are a healthier option, particularly because they contain many important vitamins (especially B complex vitamins), iron, and fiber. Examples of complex carbohydrates include dried beans and legumes like chickpeas and lentils, whole grains, fruits, and starchy vegetables like potatoes, sweet potatoes, and corn.

Try to choose whole grains over refined grains as often as possible when feeding your baby. The USDA Dietary Guidelines recommend that at least half of the grains you eat should be whole grains, so it's a good idea to start early and get your little one used to the taste of whole wheat bread and brown rice. If they get used to the taste now, there will be less chance that your child will ask for processed white bread when he or she is older. Whole grains contain all three elements of the grain: the fibrous outer portion (the bran), the inner part (the endosperm) and the heart of the grain kernel (the germ). Whole grains are packed with fiber, vitamins, minerals, and antioxidants that are beneficial for your baby's health. Refined grains like white bread, white pasta, and white rice, on the other hand, are milled. This process yields a product with a lighter texture and longer shelf life, but strips away the most nutritious parts of the grain (including fiber).

Reading Whole Grain Food Labels

Labels can be confusing. To help identify products made mostly from whole grains, look for the word "whole" before the name of the grain (example "whole wheat flour"). If this is the first ingredient listed on the label, then the product is most likely made from mostly whole grain. "Wheat flour" simply means it was made from wheat, not whole wheat.

You can also try looking for the "Whole Grain Stamp." In 2005, the Whole Grains Council created an official packaging symbol to help consumers identify real whole grain products. This 100% stamp guarantees that the food contains a full serving or more of a whole grain in each serving of that product, and that all of the grain is whole grain. The basic Whole Grain Stamp means that a product contains at least half a serving of whole grain per serving. Note that, while the labels are becoming more widely used, they are not on all products.

Fiber is important for maintaining bowel regularity and preventing constipation in your little one. But keep in mind that you should not feed your baby a high fiber diet, as too much fiber can fill your baby up before he or she has taken in all of the required nutrients. Excess fiber can also interfere with the absorption of valuable minerals and cause diarrhea.

> ## Good Carbohydrate Sources for Baby and Toddler
>
> ♥ Breast milk or formula
> ♥ Fresh fruit and vegetables
> ♥ Beans and other legumes
> ♥ Whole grains (bread, oatmeal, pasta, rice, etc.)
> ♥ Dairy products (yogurt and cheese)
> ♥ Nut and seed butters or pastes

Fueling Fats

As adults, we're often taught to avoid fat at all costs; however, your baby absolutely needs fat—and a lot of it. To give you a better idea, between 40–50 percent of the calories provided by breast milk and infant formula come from fats. Not only are fats a major energy source for your baby, but they serve as important building blocks for their hormones and cell membranes. They are also necessary for your baby's body to absorb the important fat-soluble vitamins (vitamins A, D, E, and K). And, they are essential for insulating the nerves located in your baby's brain, spinal cord, and throughout his or her body.

As with sugars, the key is in choosing the *right* fats. Unsaturated fats, which are generally considered the healthiest, are categorized as either monounsaturated or polyunsaturated. These fats are found in foods like olive oil, safflower oil, canola oil, avocados, nuts, seeds, and cold-water fish. *Saturated fats* have primarily animal origins; common sources include butter, cheese, milk, cream, meat, and poultry.

While adults should limit the amount of saturated fat in their diets, for babies things are different. The truth is that the fat in breast milk is actually composed of about 44 percent saturated fat. It's best not to limit the amount of saturated fat in your baby's diet for their first two years (unless instructed to do so by your doctor). These fats serve important functions, and many of the foods containing these saturated fats (like meat and cheese) also contain protein, vitamins, and minerals that are important for a growing baby. Rather, as your child grows up, gradually lower the amount of saturated fat in their diet. After age two, you can start transitioning to reduced-fat products. This will help lower your child's risk of developing heart disease, diabetes, and obesity as they progress into adolescence and adulthood. It also simplifies matters in that the same products can then be used for the whole family.

Trans-fats, on the other hand, should be avoided by babies. Trans-fats are a man-made fat and are the result of a process called hydrogenation, which modifies unsaturated fats to make them more stable. Trans-fats increase the shelf life of packaged foods but are bad for your body. They are found in products like margarine, vegetable shortening, French fries and other fast foods, as well as many products on grocery shelves like cookies, cakes, crackers, and granola bars. Read the nutrition labels: if you see the term *partially hydrogenated* in the ingredients list, then that tells you the product contains trans-fat.

A specific group of fats that are vital to the growth and development of your baby are the *omega-3 fatty acids*. DHA (docosahexaenoic acid) in particular is essential for the development of your baby's brain and eyes for the first few years of life. Omega-3 fatty acids are not produced by our bodies, so they must be consumed in the diet. The main food sources of DHA and EPA (eicosapentaenoic acid) are fish and fish oil, with wild salmon being especially high in omega-3s. ALA (alpha-linolenic acid), another omega-3 fatty acid, is found in many plant sources like flaxseed and flaxseed oil, canola oil, olive oil, soybeans, tofu, walnuts, pumpkin seeds, dark green, leafy vegetables, and seaweed. ALA hasn't been shown to be as powerful a health modulator as the two omega-3s found in fish—while our bodies convert ALA to DHA and EPA, the exact amount of conversion is unknown and varies from person to person, depending on a number of factors. There are many new products available now that are enriched with omega-3s, like eggs, milk, orange juice, peanut butter, cereals, oils, pasta, and other products.

Good Fat Sources for Baby and Toddler

- ❤ Breast milk or formula
- ❤ Avocado
- ❤ Fish
- ❤ Meat and poultry
- ❤ Eggs
- ❤ Dairy products (full fat)
- ❤ Oils (olive, safflower, canola, sunflower, soy)
- ❤ Nut butters

Micronutrients

Vital Vitamins

Our bodies cannot function without vitamins, which help all of our body's systems to work better. There are 13 vitamins that our bodies need: A, C, D, E, K, and the eight B vitamins. Each of these vitamins have important roles, and they all work together to help support your baby's growth and development. Rather than focusing on each individual vitamin, the important thing is to make sure your baby is getting a wide variety of nutritious food, and thus a wide variety of vitamins.

It's also important to make sure that your baby's body can make proper use of the vitamins you feed them. Some vitamins are fat-soluble, and others are water-soluble. Vitamins A, D, E and K are fat-soluble, which means that they dissolve in fat. It also means that they're stored in your body's tissues for a long time. In other words, if your child decides not to eat certain vegetables from time to time, they will survive on the fat-soluble vitamins they've already stored up. Water-soluble vitamins (vitamin C and the B vitamins) on the other hand, dissolve in water, and are not stored in the body for very long, so it's more important that your baby gets a steady daily intake of these vitamins. The water-soluble vitamins, especially vitamin C, also tend to be more fragile and can be weakened or destroyed during cooking. Certain cooking methods, like boiling, destroy nutrients more than others and should generally be avoided. It's preferable to steam or roast your fruits and vegetables when making homemade baby food, rather than boiling them (read more about this in Chapter 6).

VITAMINS AND THEIR FUNCTIONS

Vitamin:	Functions:	Found In:
Vitamin A	Important for healthy eyes, teeth and skin, as well as cell growth and a strong immune system	Yellow-orange fruits and vegetables (sweet potatoes, carrots, cantaloupe, apricots, winter squash), leafy green vegetables (kale, collards, spinach) and broccoli; eggs, meat (especially liver), milk, cheese
B Vitamins	Wide variety of functions in the body; help convert the food you eat into energy	Whole grains, fish, eggs, meat, poultry, dairy products, leafy green vegetables, and legumes
Vitamin C	Boosts your immune system, helps fight off infections, keeps your skin healthy and is essential for tissue repair and wound healing	Citrus fruit, bell peppers, strawberries, kiwi, mango, tomatoes, broccoli, cauliflower, sweet potatoes, and leafy greens
Vitamin D	Works with calcium to help build your baby's bones and teeth; often referred to as the "sunshine vitamin" because our bodies make it naturally from skin exposure to the sun	Fatty fish like salmon, tuna, sardines; and mackerel; egg yolks; cereals, milk, dairy products, and juice
Vitamin E	Powerful antioxidant that protects your cells from damage by free radicals	Nuts, seeds, avocado, tomatoes, leafy green vegetables, wheat germ, vegetable oils; cereals, juices, and spreads
Vitamin K	Essential for normal blood clotting; also important for bone health	Leafy green vegetables like kale, collard greens, spinach, beet greens, and romaine lettuce, Brussels sprouts, broccoli, cauliflower, cabbage; fish, meat, eggs, cereal

Mighty Minerals
Iron

Iron is one of the most important minerals for your developing baby's health. Iron is essential for making hemoglobin, the protein in our red blood cells that carries oxygen to our organs and tissues. Your doctor will check your baby's hemoglobin level during a well-baby checkup, usually at about 12 months (premature babies are checked earlier, usually at about 6 months). When your baby's hemoglobin level is low, it is called *anemia*. If the anemia is due to insufficient iron, the condition is called *iron-deficiency anemia*.

Iron deficiency is the most common known form of nutritional deficiency, and is most prevalent in young children and women of childbearing age. Iron deficiency during infancy increases the risk of cognitive, motor, and behavioral deficits, which can have long-term effects.

Healthy, full-term babies are usually born with enough iron stores to last them for approximately their first 4–6 months of life. They get this iron from their mothers during the last trimester of pregnancy, and they store it in their tissues and red blood cells. Pre-term babies, however, don't have enough time to build up these iron stores, and thus, are not born with such a large iron reserve.

Babies at risk for iron deficiency include:

- ✿ Babies who were born prematurely
- ✿ Babies with low birth weight
- ✿ Babies whose mothers had nutritional deficiencies like iron-deficiency anemia, or who were diabetic

In addition to the iron that your baby has stored up, your little one will be getting iron from breast milk or formula (formula is fortified with iron). Actually, breast milk does not contain particularly high levels of iron; however, infants are super efficient at absorbing iron from this source.

Once your baby starts eating solids (at about 6 months of age), they will need to be consuming about *11 mg of iron per day* (until about 12 months of age). Between the ages of 1 and 3, the requirement drops to *7 mg of iron per day*. You can help your baby to meet this requirement by feeding her or him plenty of iron-rich foods, like iron-fortified cereals, meats, grains, beans, and vegetables. Remember that your baby will also continue to absorb iron from breast milk or formula. In certain cases, if your baby is at risk for iron deficiency, your pediatrician may recommend an iron supplement. Check with your pediatrician about your baby's iron needs if you plan to make homemade cereals instead of buying iron-fortified cereal.

Good Sources of Iron

- ♥ Breast milk and iron-fortified formula
- ♥ Iron-fortified cereal (like rice, oatmeal and barley)
- ♥ Meat and poultry: beef, beef liver, lamb, chicken, chicken liver, turkey, pork, egg yolks (note that dark meat poultry has a higher iron content than white meat)
- ♥ Seafood: oysters, clams, mussels, sardines, halibut, haddock, salmon, tuna
- ♥ Legumes: white beans, kidney beans, black beans, lentils, chickpeas, tofu
- ♥ Fruits and vegetables: spinach, Swiss chard, kale, peas, beets, broccoli, sweet potatoes, dried fruit (apricots, figs, prunes, raisins), prune juice
- ♥ Grains: quinoa, amaranth, wheat germ, millet, brown rice, pasta, whole wheat bread
- ♥ Seeds (ground or mashed): sunflower, pumpkin
- ♥ Blackstrap molasses

The following are some tips to increase iron levels in your baby's diet:

Feed them a wide variety of foods that are rich in iron, including meat (unless your baby is vegetarian). There are actually two forms of iron: heme and non-heme. Plants and iron-fortified foods (like cereals, bread, and pasta) contain only the non-heme form of iron, while meat, seafood, and poultry contain both the heme and non-heme forms. The heme form of iron is much easier for your body to absorb, so vegetarians have to be careful to get enough iron in their diets.

Include foods that are rich in Vitamin C with your meals. Vitamin C greatly increases the amount of iron your body absorbs from food. Examples of good combinations include iron-fortified cereal mixed with a berry puree, chicken with apricots, and fish with peas.

Limit dairy with meals. The calcium in cow's milk actually inhibits the absorption of iron, so avoid including too much dairy with high-iron meals. You should not be giving your baby cow's milk before 12 months anyway, but when you feed him or her yogurt and cheese, try giving it as a snack between meals.

Calcium

We have more calcium in our bodies than any other mineral; 99 percent of it is stored in our bones and teeth to help make them strong. Because children are constantly growing new bones, they need a steady supply of calcium to support that growth. The remaining calcium is distributed throughout our blood and tissues, where it works to perform several vital functions, including maintaining a normal heartbeat, contracting muscles, transmitting nerve impulses and clotting of blood. Vitamin D also helps the body absorb calcium, so make sure your baby is getting enough Vitamin D.

Breast milk or formula will supply all of the calcium needed by your baby in its first year. Breast milk is actually lower in calcium than formula but, as with iron, your baby more easily absorbs the calcium in breast milk. After 1 year, cow's milk can supply your baby with plenty of calcium, as well as many other nutrients, including healthy fats, protein, and Vitamin D.

Good sources of calcium are listed in the box below. (Calcium is also added to many foods, like orange juice, plant-based milks (soy, almond, and rice milks), tofu, ready-to-eat cereals and breads.)

Good Sources of Calcium

- ♥ Milk (after 1 year), yogurt, and cheese
- ♥ Spinach, broccoli, collard greens, kale, mustard greens, and bok choy
- ♥ Dried fruit, like apricots, plums (prunes), and raisins
- ♥ Canned fish, like sardines and salmon
- ♥ Dried beans and other legumes
- ♥ Nut and seed butters and pastes like almond, peanut, or sunflower seed butter and sesame paste
- ♥ Fortified foods: orange juice, tofu, cereals, and breads

The Vegetarian Baby

Approximately 5 percent of the U.S. population follows a vegetarian diet, and that number keeps growing. In addition, many people are beginning to eat more vegetarian-style meals, even if they don't follow a completely vegetarian diet. Raising a baby on a vegetarian or vegan diet is a personal choice, and you have to choose what's best for you and your family. It can be just as healthy an option for your baby as it is for you—you just have to make sure that your baby gets the proper nutrients. It's easy to come up short on certain nutrients, so it may be a good idea to discuss a feeding plan with your doctor or a registered dietician to make sure that your baby is receiving all of the nutrients needed during this critical time when so much growth and development is taking place.

Some of the important nutrients that may be challenging to get enough of are: *protein, iron, zinc, vitamin D, vitamin B12 and omega-3 fatty acids*. Fortunately, there are plenty of vegetarian sources for most of these nutrients; the exception is vitamin B12, which is only found in animal products. The body requires a source of vitamin B12, which is essential for development of the nervous system and production of red blood cells. Some foods, like breakfast cereals, nutritional yeasts, meat substitutes, and soy milk, are fortified with vitamin B12. Formula is also supplemented with vitamin B12, but for breast-fed babies, the level of B12 in breast milk will depends on mom's diet. If your baby is vegetarian or vegan, be sure to discuss the possibility of a vitamin supplement with your doctor.

Most people tend to think of meat and dairy products when the word protein is mentioned. The fact is, protein is also found in a number of vegetarian foods, such as grains, nuts, and legumes (like beans and lentils). It's important for vegetarians to consume a wide variety of protein sources to ensure that they get all of the essential amino acids. There are some vegetarian foods like soy, quinoa, and chia seeds that are complete proteins, so keep these stocked in your kitchen (see the table on page 29 for a list of foods that are rich in protein).

Zinc is another mineral that's crucial for your baby's growth and development, specifically because it's involved in the synthesis of DNA; infants and toddlers should be getting 3 grams of zinc per day. Similar to iron, plant-based sources of zinc are not absorbed as well as animal sources, so vegetarians must be sure to increase their intake of zinc-rich foods. Good vegetarian sources of zinc are wheat germ, fortified breakfast cereals, whole grains, dairy products, nut butters, beans, green peas, and tofu.

Vitamin D is another important nutrient. Your baby's body requires an adequate amount of vitamin D in order to properly absorb calcium and phosphorus, which are essential for bone formation. Inadequate levels of vitamin D in babies can lead to a condition known as rickets, which causes bones to be fragile and to break easily. Babies should receive 400 IU of vitamin D per day, while toddlers need 600 IU. There are relatively few natural food sources of vitamin D; the best sources are fatty fish and products that are fortified with vitamin D, like cereals, milk, dairy products, and orange juice. Sun exposure is another way to increase your baby's vitamin D levels, as our bodies produce vitamin D after our skin is exposed to sunshine. Formula is also supplemented with vitamin D; however, only small amounts of vitamin D are transferred through breast milk. For this reason, your doctor may recommend a vitamin D supplement, especially if your baby is breast-fed or consumes less than 32 ounces of formula per day.

DHA, which is the most crucial omega-3 fatty acid for your baby's brain and eye development, is found mainly in cold-water fish (though DHA is also added to infant formula). Breast-fed babies may be at risk for deficiency because the amount of DHA in breast milk is proportional to the amount the mother is currently consuming. If you or your baby is vegetarian or vegan, speak to your doctor about the possibility of taking a supplement. Once your child is older, you can introduce other, non-fish sources of omega-3s, like ground flaxseeds, flaxseed oil, chia seeds, and walnuts.

To sum things up, it's important to provide your baby with a well-balanced diet in order to fuel the substantial amount of growth and development that occurs during this time. Don't worry too much about hitting the mark every single day; nutrition is about averages, so just try to provide your baby with a wide variety of foods, full of the main nutritional building blocks. Remember, you're widening their culinary horizons *and* putting them on the path to lifelong good health!

CHAPTER 5

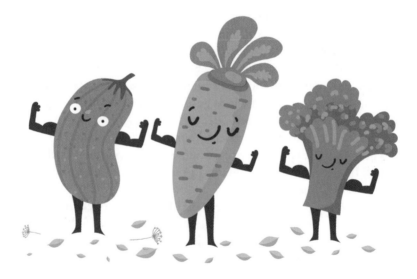

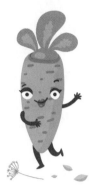

Safely Feeding Your Baby

Food Allergies: The Changing Times

The topic of food allergies is one that can often be confusing and stress-inducing for new parents. Over the past decade, the prevailing beliefs about when to introduce highly allergenic foods into your baby's diet have undergone a dramatic shift. Traditionally, the common practice in pediatrics was to delay the introduction of highly allergenic foods, based on the belief that this would prevent the development of food allergies and other atopic conditions, like eczema and allergic rhinitis. In the past, parents were told to delay giving highly allergenic foods until 12 months (cow's milk, dairy), 24 months (eggs), or even 36 months (fish, tree nuts, peanuts).

Then, in 2008, the American Academy of Pediatrics (AAP) changed its previous guidelines on the matter. They acknowledged that there was insufficient evidence to support the delayed introduction of allergens as a strategy to reduce the risk of food allergies. In fact, it turns out that delaying exposure to certain foods might actually do more harm than good. As more research becomes available, the body of evidence is starting to point in a consistent direction—that early introduction of common food allergens is associated with a lower risk of developing food allergies (compared to delayed introduction). In 2013, the American Academy of Asthma, Allergy and Immunology (AAAAI) released a study on infant feeding practices to help prevent food allergies. These recommendations are based on the available observational research to date, and are the first guidelines to state that delaying introduction of foods like wheat, cow's milk dairy, eggs, fish, and nuts may actually result in an *increased* risk of food allergy or eczema. The guidelines state that highly allergenic complementary foods may be introduced *between 4 and 6 months of age, once a few typical complementary foods have been fed and tolerated.*

What that means is that if your infant is not at high risk for allergy—once they've tolerated a few non-allergenic foods (like apples, bananas, sweet potatoes, and cereals)—you can start introducing more allergenic foods (the exception to this is cow's milk, which is still not recommended until your baby's first birthday). Ideally, you want to introduce new foods at home, rather than in a day care or restaurant setting. It's also preferable to introduce them early in the day, so that you can observe for signs of a reaction. And as with all solids, follow the 3–5 day rule to help isolate triggers of an allergic reaction. If your baby shows signs of having an allergy to a food, hold off on giving it again and consult with your baby's doctor about when to introduce common allergens.

If your baby is high risk, or has already been diagnosed with food allergies or severe eczema, then you will need to speak with your child's doctor before introducing these foods. An infant is considered to be at "high risk" for developing allergic disease if there is at least one first-degree relative (parent or sibling) with an allergic condition, including a documented food allergy, asthma, allergic rhinitis, or atopic dermatitis (eczema). If your baby is high risk, then try to breast-feed exclusively for the first 4–6 months, as this may help decrease the risk of eczema and cow's milk allergy. If this is not possible, talk to your doctor about the possibility of using a hydrolyzed ("hypoallergenic") formula instead.

Also, bear in mind that although the guidelines have changed, some pediatricians still recommend a more cautious approach with certain foods, especially with foods like eggs, peanuts, and shellfish, because of the strong allergic reactions that can be associated with them. Ultimately, how you introduce allergens into your baby's diet is a personal decision that you'll have to make in consultation with your baby's healthcare provider.

Food Allergy vs. Intolerance

Most of the reactions that occur in babies introduced to new foods are actually food intolerance, as opposed to a true allergy. True food allergies are less common than you might think: food allergies affect only about 2 percent of the general population, and 6–8 percent of children. (However, that number is on the rise. According to a report from the CDC, the prevalence of children with food allergies increased 18 percent from 1997 to 2007.) A true food allergy is an immune system reaction; your body reacts as though an ingredient in a particular food product is harmful and creates a defense system (antibodies) to fight it. Your body then releases chemicals, including histamine, which cause symptoms like itchy skin rash, runny nose, wheezing, vomiting, and diarrhea. The symptoms of a food allergy can range from mild to severe, and can even be life threatening in rare cases. Anaphylaxis is a severe, life-threatening allergic reaction with widespread effects on the body.

Signs and Symptoms of a Food Allergy

- Skin: hives (red, swollen itchy areas on the skin); eczema (itchy, dry rash); itching and swelling of the face, tongue, and mouth; redness and swelling of the face or extremities
- Gastrointestinal tract: vomiting, diarrhea, stomach pain
- Respiratory tract: runny or stuffy nose, sneezing, throat tightness, coughing, wheezing, difficulty breathing
- Cardiovascular: chest pain, lightheadedness, pale skin, fainting

If your child develops signs of a severe allergic reaction, such as swelling of the face, tongue, or lips; difficulty breathing, coughing, wheezing; or turning blue, get help immediately. Call 911 or go to the closest emergency room.

Thankfully, these types of reactions can be largely avoided by avoiding common allergy triggers. Eight types of food account for over 90 percent of allergic reactions in affected individuals: milk, eggs, peanuts, tree nuts, fish, shellfish, soy, and wheat. Although certain foods are more likely to cause problems, any food can trigger a food allergy or adverse reaction. The only way to manage allergies is to strictly avoid the offending food.

Foods Most Likely to Cause an Allergic Reaction

- Cow's milk
- Eggs
- Peanuts
- Tree nuts
- Fish
- Shellfish
- Soy
- Wheat

Food intolerance, on the other hand, does not involve the immune system. It occurs when something in a food irritates a person's digestive system, or when a person is unable to properly digest, or break down, the food. Intolerance to lactose, which is a sugar found in milk and other dairy products, is the most common food intolerance. Food intolerance can cause symptoms like diarrhea, bloating, and gas, and is often mistaken for a food allergy. Food intolerance can be unpleasant, but is rarely dangerous.

Signs and Symptoms of Food Intolerance

- Nausea or vomiting
- Diarrhea
- Gas, cramps or bloating
- Stomach pain
- Irritability or nervousness
- Headaches

If your child appears to have a reaction to a particular food, be sure to discuss it with your doctor. Usually, a careful review of the circumstances and some confirmatory testing can determine the cause. If the symptoms are persistent (or the cause is unclear), your doctor may suggest eliminating suspect foods for a period of time to see if your baby's symptoms improve. Often, a food will be tolerated well after such a period of time once your baby's digestive tract and immune system have had more time to mature. In certain cases, your doctor may refer you to a pediatric allergist for skin or blood tests. Sometimes, allergies can't be confirmed by these tests and it may be recommended that your child have a *food challenge* test, during which your baby will eat foods gradually, under the doctor's supervision.

The good news about food allergies and sensitivities is that many children outgrow them in early childhood. According to the American Academy of Pediatrics, 80–90 percent of egg, milk, wheat, and soy allergies go away by age 5. Some allergies, however, are more persistent; for example, only 1 in 5 young children will outgrow a peanut allergy, and fewer still will outgrow allergies to nuts or seafood.

Preventing Choking

Once you begin feeding your baby solids, choking becomes a real concern. Enthusiastic babies may try to stuff their mouths with the foods that they like, which can cause choking accidents. There are steps that you can take to prevent choking, but it's also important to be prepared and know what to do if your child is choking. Most community hospitals offer basic first aid and CPR classes. You can also contact your local American Red Cross, YMCA, or American Heart Association chapter to find a class in your area. These classes are a must, not only for parents, but also for anyone watching your baby, like grandparents or baby sitters.

Follow these basic guidelines to minimize your baby's risk of choking:

- Never leave your baby alone when he's eating; always keep a close eye on him
- Keep babies seated for all meals and snacks; don't allow them to run around with food in their mouths
- Keep all items that your baby could potentially choke on out of reach
- Put only a few pieces of food on their plate at a time
- When your baby is ready for finger foods, cut the food into pieces no larger than ¼ inch

There are certain foods that are dangerous and should not be given to your child due to the high risk of choking. These include:

- Hot dog pieces
- Whole nuts and seeds
- Popcorn
- Whole grapes
- Chunks of meat or cheese
- Raw vegetables
- Raisins
- Hard, gooey or sticky candy
- Sticky foods like chewing gum or marshmallows
- Chunks or large spoonfuls of nut butters (they can be spread thinly)

Choking First Aid: What To Do If Your Infant Is Conscious and Choking

(For infants 12 months and under)

- ♥ Do *not* proceed with choking first aid if your baby is coughing forcefully or has a strong cry. Wait and see if they can clear the object themselves, but be prepared to act if the symptoms worsen. Do *not* try to grasp and pull out the object if your baby is alert.

- ♥ If your baby's symptoms worsen, call 911 and begin choking first aid. If someone is with you, have them call 911 while you begin first aid. Signs that your baby may be choking are:
  - Labored breathing, with ribs and chest pulling inwards
  - Soft or high-pitched sounds when inhaling
  - Weak, ineffective coughing
  - Inability to cry

- ♥ Give five back blows. Lay your baby face down along your forearm, using your thigh or lap for support. Support the face and neck with your hand and point the head downward so that it's lower than the body. Using your free hand, give five quick, forceful blows between the shoulder blades.

- ♥ If the object does not come out of the airway after the back blows, then give five chest thrusts. To do this, turn your baby face up on your forearm, using your thigh or lap for support. Cradle their head with your hand and keep their head lower than their body. Using your free hand, place two fingers on the breastbone in middle of their chest, just below the nipple line, and give five quick thrusts down, compressing the chest about 1½ inches. Allow the chest to rise before beginning another thrust.

- ♥ Continue to repeat five back blows and five chest thrusts until the object is dislodged and your baby can cough forcefully, cry, or breathe.

- ♥ If your baby becomes unconscious, begin CPR, alternating rescue breaths and chest compressions.

Refer to the American Red Cross website (www.redcross.org) for more information.

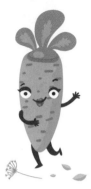

CHAPTER 6

Making Homemade Baby Food 101

Choosing Ingredients: Fruits and Vegetables

Fresh vs. Frozen

While it would seem obvious that fresh fruits and vegetables are always best, this isn't necessarily the case. Frozen fruits and vegetables are picked in season, when they're at their nutritional peak. They're also frozen soon after picking, so they don't lose many nutrients sitting around. In other words, it's best to use frozen produce for fruits and vegetables that aren't in season. It's also perfectly acceptable to use frozen fruits and vegetables for convenience's sake. Frozen fruit like mangos and pineapple are already peeled and chopped; frozen cherries are pitted, and frozen artichokes are trimmed and ready to be tossed right into your dishes. Frozen produce can also be more economical.

Canned vegetables and fruits should generally not be used too often. Canned foods go through extensive processing to make them stable enough to sit on a shelf for months or years. A lot of nutrients can be lost in the canning process because they're heated to very high temperatures. Even more nutrients can leach out into the water that they're packed in, which you usually end up throwing out. Also, many canned vegetables and fruit are high in sodium or sugar. (One notable exception is canned pumpkin, which is pureed. This convenient product is labeled as 100 percent pumpkin, with no fillers; this is different from "pumpkin pie mix" which is sweetened and has other added ingredients). If you do buy canned fruit, be sure to look for fruit labeled "packed in its own juice" or "unsweetened."

Organic vs. Conventional

Now that you're going to be making homemade baby food, you're probably wondering about the effects of pesticides on your baby's health. This is a good time to consider buying organic. This is an area with a lot of ongoing research, and we're learning more and more every day about the potentially harmful long-term effects of pesticides on our health. At the same time, the organic movement has been growing in leaps and bounds as consumers become more educated on these issues.

Babies and young children have rapidly developing brains and are uniquely vulnerable to chemical exposures. When preparing food for your baby, it makes sense to try and go organic when possible. In order for a food to be labeled "organic," it has to meet certain standards set by the U.S. Department of Agriculture (USDA). Organic food must be grown or produced without any chemical pesticides or fertilizers; livestock must be raised without the use of antibiotics or growth hormones. Organic foods also cannot be genetically modified, irradiated or cloned.

Organic produce does tend to cost more than conventional produce, but as the organic movement continues to grow, the price gap gets narrower. If you are on a budget, a good place to start would be to buy organic for those items that matter the most and to buy conventional for the rest. Each year, the Environmental Working Group, a nonprofit group, publishes a list of the fruits and vegetables with the most and least pesticide residues, which they call the "Dirty Dozen" and the "Clean Fifteen." By choosing to buy organic for the most heavily contaminated items, you can significantly decrease your intake of pesticides. Take a look at their website (www.ewg.org) and make the decision that's best for you and your family. I also suggest buying organic poultry, meat, and dairy whenever possible.

At the end of the day, the most important thing is to feed your baby a healthy diet, rich in a wide variety of fruit, vegetable, whole grains, and proteins. So don't feel bad if organic ingredients aren't in your budget. The health benefits of truly nutritious foods outweigh the potential negatives.

Buying Organic:
The "Dirty Dozen" and the "Clean Fifteen"

"Dirty Dozen" 2015
Purchase organic:

Apples	Celery	Snap peas (imported)
Peaches	Spinach	Potatoes
Nectarines	Sweet bell peppers	(also, Hot peppers,
Strawberries	Cucumbers	Kale and Collard greens)
Grapes	Cherry tomatoes	

"The Clean Fifteen" 2015
Safe to purchase conventional:

Avocados	Onions	Eggplant
Sweet corn	Asparagus	Grapefruit
Pineapple	Mangos	Cantaloupe
Cabbage	Papayas	Cauliflower
Sweet peas (frozen)	Kiwi	Sweet potatoes

A Note on Nitrates

You may have heard that you should be avoiding making certain homemade baby foods because of the high concentration of nitrates. Nitrates are chemicals found in water and soil, with some nitrates being naturally occurring and others manufactured in a lab, for use in fertilizers. Nitrate poisoning may lead to a rare condition called methemoglobinemia, also called "blue baby syndrome." This is a form of anemia that affects the ability of red blood cells to transport oxygen to the body's cells.

Nitrate levels are found in their highest concentration in well water, but some vegetables can also contain nitrates—spinach, beets, green beans, squash, and carrots being the most common examples. But the truth is that methemoglobinemia in babies is almost always caused by drinking infant formula made with well water that's been contaminated by nitrates from synthetic fertilizer, *not* by eating homemade baby food. There has only been *one* reported case: in this country, in 1973, a baby developed nitrate poisoning from home-prepared vegetable foods, when drinking too much contaminated carrot juice.

They key issue is the age of the baby. To be on the safe side, the official AAP guidelines on nitrates say: "Home-prepared infant foods from vegetables (e.g., spinach, beets, green beans, squash, and carrots) should be avoided *until infants are 3 months or older*. This is because nitrates are mostly a risk to fetal blood cells, which are almost completely gone by 3 months of age. Furthermore, by 6 months, your baby's stomach and digestive system are fully developed and can handle normal nitrate exposure from any homemade foods.

So to sum it up, this really shouldn't be an issue, provided you are already waiting to introduce solids into your baby's diet until they are at least 4–6 months—completely in line with current AAP recommendations.

To reduce your exposure, you can choose organic vegetables for these foods, as the nitrate levels will be significantly reduced (but not eliminated entirely). If you will be using well water to make your baby's food, have it tested; it should contain less than 10 ppm of nitrates.

Choosing Ingredients: Meat and Eggs

Consider buying organic for meat, poultry, and eggs—organically raised animals are not given any antibiotics or hormones. Meat from grass-fed, organically raised cattle tends to be leaner and has higher levels of omega-3s. Also, when the label indicates DHA-enhanced eggs (sometimes called omega-3 eggs), it means the eggs were laid by chickens on a vegetarian, DHA-supplemented diet.

When purchasing meat and poultry, give the items a quick visual inspection before purchasing them. Red meat should have a bright red color and be firm to the touch; try to buy lean cuts of meat, and avoid cuts that look gray or fatty. Raw chicken should have a pink color, and should not also look gray or slimy.

Seafood

Fish and shellfish are rich in omega-3 fatty acids, protein, vitamins, and minerals, and can be a healthy addition to your baby's diet. Omega-3 fatty acids are crucial for the development of your baby's brain and vision, and seafood is one of the best sources of this nutrient. However, certain types of fish can contain potentially harmful levels of mercury that can affect your baby's developing nervous system. The amount of contaminants depends on the type of fish and where it's caught. Every state issues advisories about the safe amount of locally caught fish that can be consumed. Alaskan seafood in particular is among the purest in the world—Alaska's marine habitats are nearly pollution free, which produces fish with superior flavor and texture. Alaskan seafood is also an environmentally responsible choice, as its fisheries are managed for sustainability.

When you feed your baby fish, be sure to avoid high-mercury fish such as swordfish, shark, king mackerel, and tilefish (you should also limit the amount of tuna). Instead, enjoy low-mercury seafood like salmon, shrimp, pollock, tilapia, catfish, and cod.

When buying fresh seafood, do a quick visual examination and smell test before purchasing. Seafood should not smell fishy if it's fresh; it should smell like the ocean. Live shellfish like mussels and clams should have closed shells; if they're open, discard them.

Getting Started in the Kitchen

Before we get started with the recipes, we'll go over the basic steps for preparing baby food at home: *Prep, Cook, Puree, Serve,* and *Store.* First, here's a list of some common kitchen equipment that you'll likely need for each step. While there are dedicated baby food makers on the market that steam and puree your food all in one, you don't need to get one just to make your own baby food. Instead, all you need is a few items, many of which you may already have in your kitchen.

Kitchen Equipment:
- For Prep:
  - Cutting boards (one for meat and one for everything else)
  - Chef's knife
  - Small paring knife
  - Kitchen shears
  - Measuring cups and spoons
- For Cooking:
  - Medium or large saucepan
  - Steamer basket
  - Baking sheet
  - Muffin tin
- For Pureeing:
  - Blender (traditional or immersion) or
  - Food processor (regular size or mini)
  - Food mill or ricer
  - Potato masher or fork
  - Strainer
- For Serving:
  - Bowls
  - Soft-tipped spoons
  - Bibs
  - Splash mat
- For Storing:
  - Ice cube trays or other airtight food storage containers
  - Freezer bags
  - Marker for labeling

Prep

Wash your produce thoroughly! This includes fruits and vegetables with skin and rinds that won't be eaten. This is important, as the bacteria living on the surface of produce can get transferred to the rest of the fruit/vegetable when you cut into it or peel it. Peel and then cut food into uniform pieces. This will help it to cook evenly.

Cooking

Cook in large batches to save time. If you set aside a few hours one day, you can make enough baby food to last for weeks. If you're turning on the oven to cook dinner for the family, throw in a bunch of vegetables for your baby's food, too.

In general, when making baby food, steaming and roasting are the preferred methods (poaching is also a good option for meat and fish). Try to avoid boiling for the most part, as boiling can leach a lot of important nutrients into the water. In fact, fruits and vegetables can lose as much as 50 percent of their vitamins, minerals, and antioxidants when boiled, which is the last thing you want when preparing food for your baby. The longer you cook them, the more nutrients are lost. Also, boiling can significantly alter the taste, color, and texture of the food—we've all had bland, mushy, colorless peas that have been cooked to death!

Steaming

Steaming is a moist-heat cooking technique in which hot steam cooks the food. Food retains most of its nutrients with steaming because it does not come into contact with the water. Steaming is the method of choice for cooking fruits and vegetables (it can also be used for fish). Cut the food you're steaming into uniformly sized pieces so that they cook in the same amount of time. Add 1 inch of water to a saucepan and insert a steamer basket. The surface of the water should be lower than the basket, and should not be touching it at all (pour some water out if needed). Bring the water to a boil. Once you start to see steam emerging from the pot, add your food to the steamer basket. Cover the pot with a tight lid and reduce the heat to medium, so that the water is simmering. The food is done when it can be easily pierced with a knife. For foods that take a long time to steam (like squash or sweet potatoes), keep an eye on the water level as you may need to replenish it. Carefully remove the food and cool slightly before pureeing. Always be careful when opening the steamer and taking the food out, as the steam is very hot!

Roasting

Roasting uses the hot, dry heat of the oven to cook food. It also browns and caramelizes the surface of the food while concentrating the natural sugars in fruits and vegetables, intensifying the flavors. It takes more time than some other cooking methods, but it's hands-off.

Once you pop your food in the oven you can do something else (like take a much-needed nap!) Roasting is a great choice for starchy vegetables like potatoes, sweet potatoes, squash, pumpkin, and beets, as well as for fruits like apples, peaches, plums, and apricots. Roasting is also an excellent choice for cooking meat, poultry or fish, which remain moist and juicy. To roast, line a baking sheet with parchment paper or foil and place the food you're cooking on top of it. The recipe may call for brushing the food with oil or adding seasonings, after which you can just pop the whole thing in the oven. The temperature and time depend on what you're cooking. Always cook meat and seafood fully when making baby food (refer to the Food Temperature Guide on page 55). Use a meat thermometer if there's any question.

Let meat rest before cutting it into pieces and pureeing. Fish can usually be flaked with a fork and mashed or pureed. Always use oven mitts when handling hot food and kitchen equipment.

Poaching

Poaching is a versatile cooking technique that involves simmering food in a liquid (like water or stock) in a pan on the stove. It's a good option for cooking fish, as well as chicken. It produces a very moist, evenly cooked product. You can flavor the poaching liquid by adding herbs and spices. Reserve the cooking liquid to add to the food when you're pureeing it.

Stewing

Stewing is a long, slow method of cooking that involves putting pieces of fruit, vegetable, or meat into a heavy-bottomed pot with a little water (if necessary), and then covering and cooking over low heat until soft. It's used in dishes like applesauce and beef stew.

Pureeing

Once the food is cooked, you then have to puree it. How smooth a puree you make depends on the stage your baby is at. In the beginning, your purees will be totally smooth, but as your little one grows and develops, you will want to leave them chunkier. Below are some options for kitchen equipment that you can use to puree your baby food.

Blender

The blender is easy, quick, and purees to a smooth consistency. Make sure that when using a blender you let the food cool slightly before blending; otherwise, the steam from the hot food can cause the lid to pop off. It's a good idea to remove the plastic insert from the blender top and hold a towel over the top as you blend. This reduces the pressure inside the blender so that your kitchen doesn't end up a spattered mess. Add a small amount of water, breast milk, or formula to the blender as needed to help the puree blend smoothly, and scrape down the sides frequently.

Some parents may want to consider an immersion blender, which is a type of handheld blender that can be used directly in the cooking pot. This results in fewer dishes, which is a huge plus. Immersion blenders can be used for making small amounts of purees, and are also great for making soup. They work best for soft foods like ripe fruits and cooked vegetables. They are not so good for meat, poultry, beans, or starchy vegetables like potatoes.

Food Processor
Easy, quick, and equipped with a variety of blades, standard food processors are good for bulk preparations, while mini food processors are better for smaller amounts. Food processors puree well, but usually will not get as smooth as a blender. As your baby gets older, you can pulse food in a food processor for a coarser, chunkier texture.

Food Mill or Ricer
A manual device, a food mill or ricer requires a little more muscle to use. They are good for starchy vegetables like potatoes, which may get gummy in a blender or food processor, Food mills are also good for pureeing foods that have a tough skin, because you can discard the hard parts.

Potato Masher or Fork
Quick and inexpensive, potato mashers are best for naturally soft foods. They work well as your baby gets older and can tolerate lumpier textures. If you don't have one, you can always use a good old fork!

Strainer
With your baby's first fruit and vegetable purees, you may need to strain certain recipes to remove all the lumps and get it completely smooth. Push the puree through the strainer with the back of a spoon. This will also catch any seeds or tough fibers.

Serving
Place the desired amount of baby food in a small bowl to serve, making sure the temperature and consistency are okay. Don't serve the food directly from a large container of food if you plan to use it again; the spoon will transfer bacteria from your baby's mouth to the food, so whatever portion they don't eat should be thrown away. To minimize waste, it's a good idea to put just a small portion of food in a bowl. You can always heat up more, but you can't put it back. Have a bib and splash mat ready!

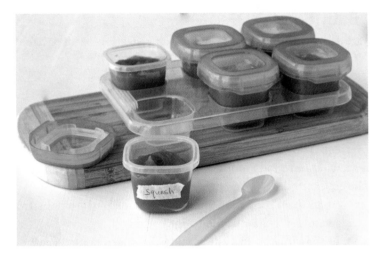

Storing

A general rule of thumb is that most baby food can be stored in the fridge for up to 3 days or in the freezer for up to 3 months. Certain purees do not freeze well (like melon, cucumber, and citrus fruit) so these foods should be made in small batches.

To store in the fridge, portion your food into clean, empty baby food jars or other individual serving containers with lids.

To store in the freezer, you can portion your food into ice cube trays or multi-portion baby food containers. Both are usually 1 ounce. The advantage of ice cube trays is that you may already have them to hand. Several brands make baby food containers for the freezer, many of which are made of silicone, which makes it easy to pop the frozen cubes out without having to warm the tray first. They also usually come with secure lids that prevent freezer burn, so for small batches of food you can store them safely in these containers. Whatever type of tray you're using, if you're making a large batch of food, pop the cubes out once the food is frozen and store them in airtight freezer bags.

Another option is to freeze portions of baby food in mounds or dollops on a cookie sheet, much like you would when baking cookies. Place dollops of pureed food (about 1 ounce or 2 tablespoons each) on a baking sheet lined with wax paper. Once frozen, transfer the frozen portions to freezer bags. The downside of this method is that it requires a lot of freezer space.

No matter which method you use, always be sure to label each bag with the type of food, as well as the date; this is very important to keep track of how old your food is.

Reheating Baby Food

The following are some basic rules to follow when reheating leftover baby food for your little one:

- ✿ Most purees should be served warm or at room temperature. Thaw out different ingredients so that you can make yummy combinations!
- ✿ Throw away any refrigerated baby food that hasn't been used after three days. Never refreeze baby food that's already been defrosted.
- ✿ When thawing out food from the freezer, never thaw at room temperature, such as on the countertop.
- ✿ The best way to thaw baby food is to move the desired portions from the freezer to the fridge and let it thaw in the fridge overnight.
- ✿ You can also thaw frozen food by placing the sealed container of food in a warm water bath.
- ✿ You can run the container of food under hot water to loosen it and then warm it in a saucepan with a little water over medium-low heat

If you're pressed for time, you can thaw food in the microwave, although this is sometimes not recommended because it heats the food unevenly. Food may feel cool on the outside while the inner temperatures are scorching hot. If you do thaw in the microwave, be very cautious. Place the frozen puree cube in a microwave-safe dish and use the defrost setting. Be sure to stir the food thoroughly to get rid of any hot spots. Always check the temperature of the food before giving it to your baby. The food should be warm but not too hot; baby's mouths are more sensitive to heat than ours are.

Food Safety

Proper sanitation and hygiene are essential when preparing food for your baby. There are four basic steps to food safety—*Clean, Separate, Cook,* and *Chill.*

Clean: Wash hands and surfaces often. Bacteria and viruses can live all over your kitchen, in places like your cutting board, sink, countertops, and utensils, as well as on your hands. These bacteria can then be transferred to your baby's food without your realizing it. To help prevent the spread of harmful bacteria, wash your hands with soap and running water before and after handling food. Wash your produce, including fruits and vegetables with skin and rinds that are not eaten. Wash cutting boards, utensils, dishes, and countertops with hot soapy water after the preparation of any raw poultry, meat, or seafood products and before preparing any other food items. When cleaning up juices from meat, poultry, or seafood, it's best to use paper towels and throw them away, as bacteria love to grow on sponges and damp dishtowels.

Separate: Don't cross-contaminate. Cross-contamination occurs when bacteria and viruses are transferred from one food to another. This is especially dangerous with raw meat, poultry, seafood, and eggs. To avoid cross-contamination, separate these items from other food items in your shopping cart, grocery bags, and refrigerator. Use two separate cutting boards—one solely for raw meat and one for ready-to-serve foods like fruits, vegetables, breads, and cooked meat.

Cook: Cook food to a safe temperature. The bacteria that cause food poisoning multiply fastest between 40°F and 140°F, which is why this temperature range is referred to as the *danger zone*. It's important to make sure that meat is cooked all the way through when making food for your baby. This will kill any harmful bacteria. The best way to make sure that your food is cooked to the proper temperature is to use a food thermometer. The table below lists the recommended safe minimum internal temperatures for meat, poultry, seafood, and egg products.

FOOD TEMPERATURE GUIDE

These are the USDA-FDA recommended safe minimum internal temperatures. Use a food thermometer to be most accurate.

Fish	145° F
Beef, pork, veal, lamb, steak, roasts, and chops	145° F (with a 3-minute rest time)
Ground beef, pork, veal, and lamb	160° F
Egg dishes	160° F
Turkey, chicken, and duck (including ground)	165° F

Chill: Refrigerate promptly. Just as cooking food at high temperatures helps kill harmful bacteria, chilling food to proper temperatures is equally important for preventing foodborne illness. Remember the danger zone (40–140°F); your refrigerator should always be set at 40°F or below, because cold temperatures slow the growth of harmful bacteria. Your freezer should be set at 0°F or below. Refrigerate meat, poultry, seafood, and any other perishable items within two hours of buying them. Food should also be refrigerated within two hours of cooking. You don't need to wait for it to cool before refrigerating or freezing.

If you follow these basic food safety guidelines, you will be well on your way to ensuring your safety and the safety of your baby. Get into the habit of reading food labels when you shop for food, and check the "sell by" dates to make sure your food is not expired. Check your fridge and freezer periodically and throw away any food that is expired. When in doubt, throw it out!

Pantry Essentials

Having a well-stocked kitchen is one of the keys to making easy, healthy meals for your family. With the right ingredients, you can create delicious dishes at home without having to make last-minute runs to the grocery store. The following is a list of some of the common ingredients used throughout this cookbook. Having these items on hand will help you be prepared so that you're never stuck trying to answer the question, "What's for dinner?"

Breads, Cereals and Grains
- Iron-fortified cereals (like rice, oatmeal, and barley)
- Whole grain bread and tortillas
- Breadcrumbs (whole wheat and panko)
- Whole wheat or multigrain pasta
- Whole grain cereal (low sugar)
- Oats: old-fashioned (rolled), quick-cooking, and/or steel-cut oats
- Rice: brown, arborio
- Barley
- Quinoa
- Millet
- Polenta or grits
- Wheat germ

Baking
- Flour: all-purpose, white whole wheat and whole wheat pastry flour
- Baking powder
- Baking soda
- Vanilla extract (no alcohol) or vanilla beans
- Sugar: unrefined sugars (like coconut palm sugar or muscovado sugar) are preferred; also brown sugar and granulated white sugar
- Honey (after 1 year old)
- Maple syrup
- Molasses

Canned
- Beans: black, kidney, pinto, cannellini
- Tomatoes: whole, crushed, puree, paste
- Marinara sauce (lower sodium)
- Olives
- Roasted red peppers
- Coconut milk
- Pumpkin
- Applesauce

Oils, Seasonings and Sauces
- Olive oil
- Neutral-flavored oil (safflower, grapeseed, peanut or canola)
- Coconut oil
- Sesame oil
- Vinegar: balsamic, cider, red, white, rice
- Dijon mustard
- Barbecue sauce
- Dried spices

Nuts, Seeds and Legumes
- Flaxseed (and/or flaxseed oil)
- Chia seeds
- Nut/seed butters: almond, peanut, sunflower seed
- Lentils: red, yellow, brown, green
- Split peas
- Dried beans
- Hummus

Dairy and Soy
- Milk: cow's milk (after 1 year) or milk alternatives like soy or almond (if vegan)
- Greek yogurt
- Cheese: sliced and/or shredded
- Cottage cheese
- Ricotta cheese
- Cream cheese
- Tofu
- Unsalted butter
- Omega-3-fortified eggs

Poultry and Meat
- ✿ Seafood: low mercury fish, shrimp
- ✿ Poultry: white and dark meat cuts, ground chicken or turkey, cooked rotisserie chicken
- ✿ Meat: lean cuts of beef, lamb, and pork, ground beef

Frozen Food
- ✿ Vegetables: spinach, broccoli, edamame, mixed vegetables
- ✿ Fruit: berries, mango, peaches, pineapple, cherries
- ✿ Brown rice
- ✿ Chicken breasts
- ✿ Ground beef, chicken, or turkey
- ✿ Pizza dough
- ✿ Whole grain or sprouted bread
- ✿ Whole grain waffles or pancakes

Produce
- ✿ In-season fruits and vegetables (can buy pre-cut to save time, like butternut squash)
- ✿ Onions, leeks, and/or shallots
- ✿ Garlic
- ✿ Fresh herbs

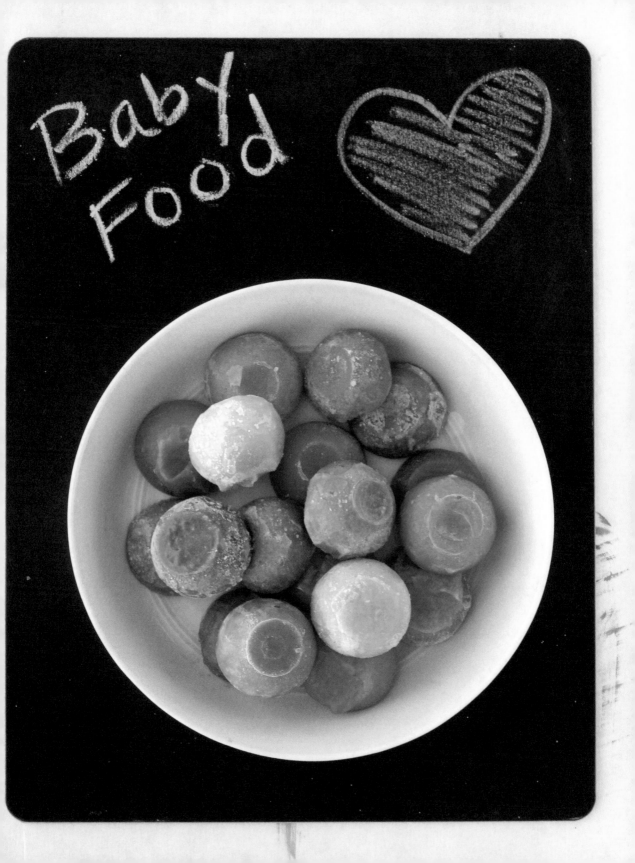

Pretty in Pink Raspberry
Pear Puree, page 108

PART II

THE
RECIPES

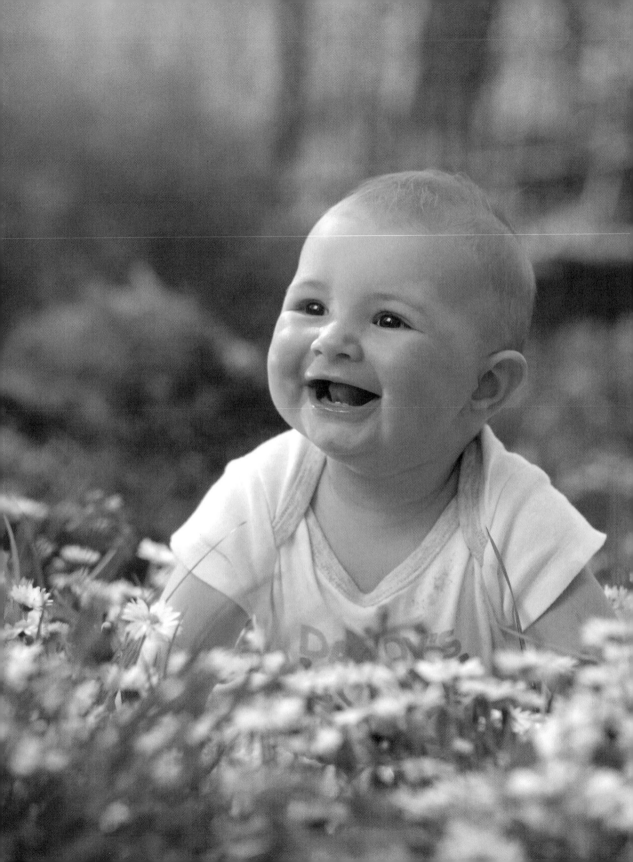

FIRST SPOONFULS: 6 MONTHS

THIS CHAPTER PROVIDES SEVERAL recipes for good "starter purees," including vegetables, fruits, and whole grain cereals. Remember that at this stage, your purees should have a thin, runny consistency. You should gradually increase the thickness over the next few months as your baby becomes more accustomed to eating solids. You can thin out your purees as needed with a little breast milk, formula, or water; or, if you need to thicken your purees, you can add a little cereal to them.

Remember to always introduce only one ingredient at a time, and to wait for 3–5 days before introducing another new food. Breast milk or formula is still your baby's primary source of nutrition at this point, and they should be eating 24–32 ounces per day. When you introduce new foods, continue to give your baby the other foods they've already been introduced to. That way, by the end of the first month, they will have been exposed to a wide variety of ingredients.

Once your baby is used to eating solids and has some experience under his or her belt, you can boost the flavor of your purees by adding some herbs and spices. Just like any other food, herbs and spices should be introduced one at a time. Suggestions for seasonings are included at the end of each puree, and are marked as "Flavor Boosts."

You can also start combining purees. At the end of the chapter are some ideas for tasty combinations to try, but feel free to create your own. As long as your baby has experience tolerating the individual components, have fun experimenting!

The sample feeding schedule below is for a baby first starting solids. With the first few feedings, try introducing solids at one meal per day. Breakfast is a good time to start so that you can observe your baby for any adverse reactions throughout the day. You want your baby to be hungry but not overly starving, so if needed, you can give them a small amount of breast milk or formula first. Start small, with about 1 tablespoon of food. Over the next several feedings, as your baby becomes accustomed to eating, you can increase the amount so that you're giving 2–4 tablespoons at a feeding. Once your baby is ready, introduce solids during a second meal in the day (like the early evening feeding). Eventually, you will work your way up to three solids meals a day (see sample menu in the next chapter).

SAMPLE FEEDING SCHEDULE FOR A BABY FIRST STARTING SOLIDS

MEAL	SAMPLE FEEDING SCHEDULE
Early morning	4–8 ounces breast milk or formula
Breakfast	1–4 tablespoons cereal, fruit or vegetable
Mid-morning	4–8 ounces breast milk or formula
Lunch	4–8 ounces breast milk or formula
Mid-afternoon	4–8 ounces breast milk or formula
Dinner	4–8 ounces breast milk or formula
Before Bed	4–8 ounces breast milk or formula

Apple Puree,
page 76

Carrot Puree,
page 72

Vegetable
Purees

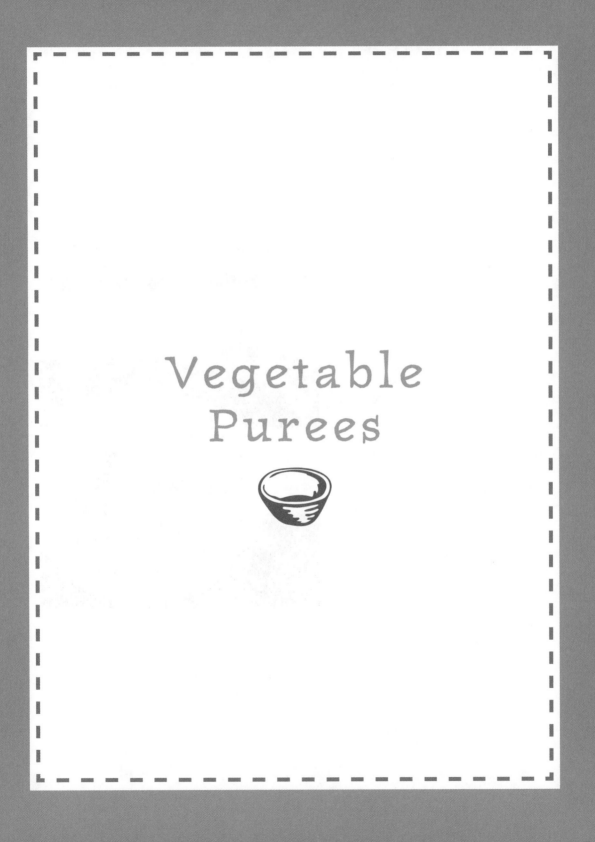

Sweet Potato Puree

Makes 2 cups

Sweet potatoes are an excellent starter food. They are nutritional superstars and babies love their sweet flavor and creamy texture. Sweet potatoes are packed with beta-carotene, a powerful anti-oxidant that gets converted to Vitamin A in the body. They're also rich in Vitamin C, Vitamin B6, fiber, manganese, and potassium. Roasting them gives them a rich flavor and there's less prep involved—no peeling and chopping. If you prefer, they can also be steamed. As your baby gets older, you can skip the pureeing step and simply mash the potatoes with a fork, leaving a little texture.

**2 large sweet potatoes,
scrubbed well**

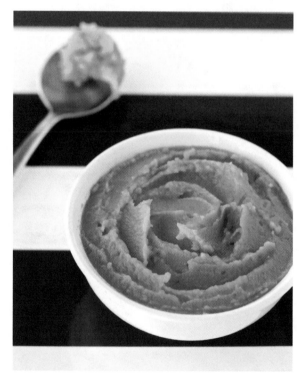

Preheat oven to 400°F.

Pierce the potatoes in several places with a fork and place them on a lined baking sheet. Roast in the oven until tender, 45–55 minutes. Remove from the oven and let cool.

Cut the potatoes in half lengthwise and scoop out the flesh with a spoon. Transfer to a food processor or blender and puree until smooth. Add a small amount of water, breast milk, or formula as needed to reach desired consistency. Serve or store.

Sweet potato puree can be stored in the refrigerator in an airtight container for 3 days or in the freezer for 3 months. If freezing, spoon individual portions into ice cube trays or baby food containers, then cover and freeze.

Steaming Method: Alternatively, you can steam the sweet potatoes instead of roasting them. To do this, peel and chop the potatoes and place them in a steamer basket set over boiling water. Cover and steam until tender, about 15 minutes. Puree as described above.

Flavor boost: cinnamon, nutmeg, cumin

Butternut Squash Puree

Makes 2 ½ cups

Butternut squash has a mild, sweet flavor that babies enjoy. It's also easy to digest and is packed with nutrients, especially Vitamins A and C. It can be roasted or steamed and if you have any leftovers, you can use it to make butternut squash soup for the rest of the family. To save time, buy pre-cut squash, which is available in most grocery stores. This recipe can also be used for other winter squash like acorn squash or pumpkin— although you may need to adjust the cooking time.

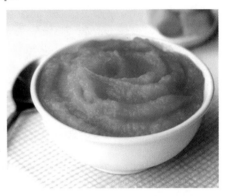

1 small butternut squash (about 1 ½ pounds)

Preheat oven to 400°F.

Trim the ends off the squash and cut it in half lengthwise. Using a spoon, scrape out the seeds and the fibrous strings from the middle.

Place the squash halves, cut side down, on a baking sheet lined with parchment paper. Roast in the oven until tender, 40–50 minutes. Remove from the oven and let cool.

Once cool, scoop out the flesh with a spoon and transfer it to a food processor or blender. Puree until smooth. Add enough water, breast milk or formula as needed to reach desired consistency. Serve or store.

Butternut squash puree can be stored in the refrigerator in an airtight container for 3 days or in the freezer for 3 months. If freezing, spoon individual portions into ice cube trays or baby food containers, then cover and freeze.

Steaming Method: Alternatively, you can steam the squash instead of roasting it. To do this, peel the squash, cut it in half and remove the seeds. Chop the squash and place the pieces in a steamer basket set over boiling water. Cover and steam until tender. Puree as described above.

Flavor boost: cinnamon, sage, thyme

Sweet Pea Puree

Makes 1½ cups

Pea puree is a great first food. It's mild, easy to digest, and has a sweet flavor that pairs well with many fruits and vegetables. Technically a legume, the humble pea is loaded with antioxidants and anti-inflammatory nutrients and is also a rich source of fiber, Vitamin A, Vitamin C, Vitamin K, folate, and iron. Take advantage of frozen peas that are picked and frozen at the height of freshness. They're just as nutritious as fresh peas and they're a whole lot easier to prepare. Besides, who has time to shell fresh peas?

1 bag (10 ounces) frozen peas

Place the peas in a steamer basket set over boiling water. Cover and steam until tender, 5–6 minutes. Remove peas from the steamer, reserving the cooking liquid.

Puree with a food processor or blender until smooth. Add a small amount of cooking liquid as needed to reach desired consistency. Cool and serve or store.

For a perfectly smooth puree, use a blender or pass the puree through a strainer to remove any solids/fibrous materials.

Pea puree can be stored in the refrigerator in an airtight container for 3 days or in the freezer for 3 months. If freezing, spoon individual portions into ice cube trays or baby food containers, then cover and freeze.

Flavor boost: mint, basil, tarragon

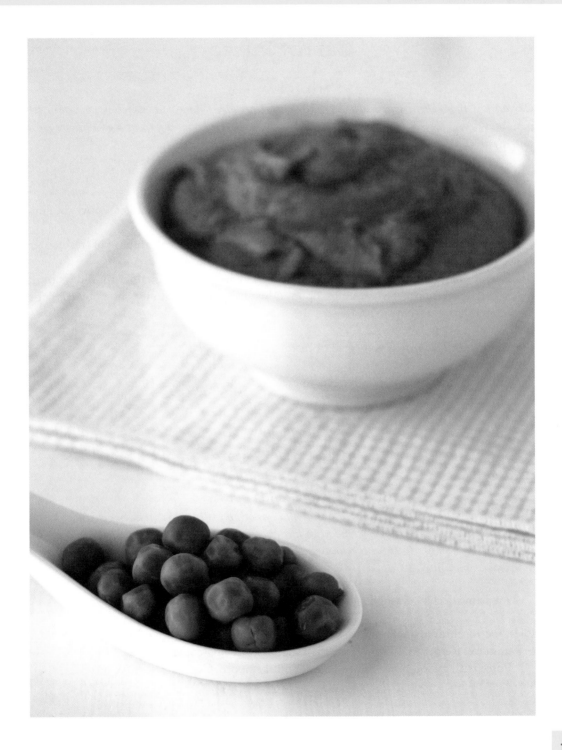

Carrot Puree

Makes 1½ cups

Carrots are an excellent source of many nutrients, especially Vitamin A, which is important for your baby's eyes. They have a mild taste and are easily digested, making them a good choice for a starter puree.

6 medium carrots (1 pound), peeled and trimmed

Cut the carrots into small pieces or slices and place them in a steamer basket set over boiling water. Cover and steam until tender, 10–12 minutes.

Puree with a food processor or blender until smooth. Add a small amount of fresh water as needed to reach desired consistency. Cool and serve or store.

Carrot puree can be stored in the refrigerator in an airtight container for 3 days or in the freezer for 3 months. If freezing, spoon individual portions into ice cube trays or baby food containers, then cover and freeze.

Parsnip Puree: Use parsnips instead of carrots

Flavor boost: cinnamon, coriander, ginger

Zucchini Puree

Makes about 2 cups

Zucchini is a good first food because it has a mild flavor and is easy to digest. In general, you can leave the skin on because it's very tender. In fact, most of the nutrients are contained in the skin, including Vitamin C. Zucchini is packed with water, so you probably won't need any additional liquid when pureeing.

2 medium zucchini, washed and sliced into ½-inch slices

Place the zucchini in a steamer basket set over boiling water. Cover and steam until tender, 6–8 minutes. Remove zucchini from the steamer, reserving cooking liquid.

Puree with a food processor or blender until smooth. Cool and serve or store.

Zucchini puree can be stored in the refrigerator in an airtight container for 3 days or in the freezer for 3 months. If freezing, spoon individual portions into ice cube trays or baby food containers, then cover and freeze.

Summer Squash Puree: Use summer squash instead of zucchini

Flavor boost: mint, basil, oregano

Potato Puree

Makes 2 cups

Although sweet potatoes tend to outshine them, white potatoes have nutritional benefits of their own, including plenty of potassium, iron, Vitamin C, and Vitamin B6. Potato puree works well in combination with other vegetable purees (like green beans) to give them a creamy texture. To keep the potatoes smooth and fluffy, use a food mill or ricer; a food processor will make the puree gummy.

2 medium potatoes (russet or Yukon Gold), washed, peeled, and chopped

Place the potato in a steamer basket set over boiling water. Cover and steam until tender, about 12–15 minutes. Remove potatoes from the steamer, reserving cooking liquid.

Run the potatoes through a food mill or ricer for a smooth puree, or mash with a potato masher or fork. Add a small amount of the cooking liquid as needed to reach desired consistency. Cool and serve or store.

Potato puree can be stored in the refrigerator in an airtight container for 3 days or in the freezer for 3 months. If freezing, spoon individual portions into ice cube trays or baby food containers, then cover and freeze.

Flavor boost: dill, parsley, rosemary

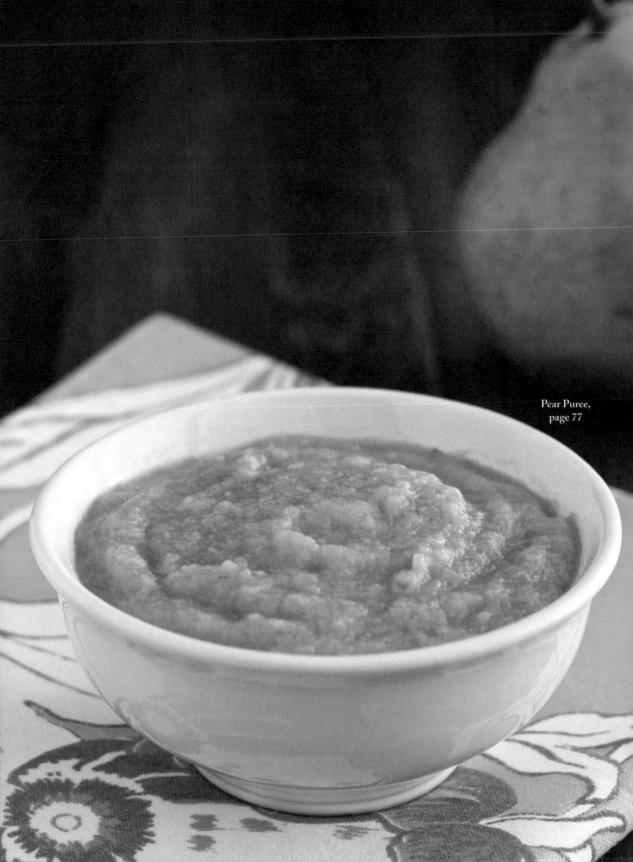

Pear Puree,
page 77

Fruit
Purees

Apple Puree

Makes 2 cups

A good source of fiber and Vitamin C, apples are mild, easy to digest, and non-allergenic, making them an excellent first food. Try to use sweet varieties of apples, like Fuji, Red, or Golden Delicious, Gala, or Honeycrisp instead of tart ones like Granny Smith. Apples consistently rank near the top of the Environmental Working Group's annual "dirty dozen list" of the fruits and vegetables with the highest pesticide residues, so try to buy organic when possible. Apple puree is one of the most versatile purees and can be mixed with a wide variety of fruits, vegetables, meat, and cereals/ grains.

4 large apples (8 ounces each), washed thoroughly

Peel, core, and chop the apples. Place the apples in a steamer basket set over boiling water. Cover and steam until tender, 10–12 minutes.

Puree with an immersion blender or food processor until smooth. Add a small amount of the cooking as needed to reach desired consistency. Cool and serve or store.

Apple puree can be stored in the refrigerator in an airtight container for 3 days or in the freezer for 3 months. Some discoloration and browning may occur with storage. If freezing, spoon individual portions into ice cube trays or baby food containers, then cover and freeze.

Flavor boost: cinnamon, nutmeg, allspice, vanilla

Pear Puree

Makes 2 cups

Pears are a good source of Vitamin C and Vitamin K, and their high fiber content works well to alleviate constipation. They have a mild, sweet flavor, are easy to digest, and are non-allergenic, which makes them a great food for young babies. Pears have a high water content, so you won't need to add any additional water when pureeing. As your baby gets older, you can skip the steaming step if you use ripe pears. Similar to apple puree, pear puree can be mixed with a wide variety of fruits, vegetables, meat, and cereals/grains.

4 large ripe pears (8 ounces each), washed thoroughly

Peel, core and chop the pears.

Place the pears in a steamer basket set over boiling water. Cover and steam until tender, 5–8 minutes.

Puree with an immersion blender or food processor until smooth. Cool and serve or store.

Pear puree can be stored in the refrigerator for 3 days or in the freezer for 3 months. Some discoloration and browning may occur with storage. If freezing, spoon individual portions into ice cube trays or baby food containers, then cover and freeze.

Flavor boost: cinnamon, cloves, ginger, rosemary

Banana Mash,
page 80

No-Cook
Purees

Banana Mash

Makes about ⅓ cup

Bananas are rich in potassium and fiber, and their sweet flavor makes them very versatile. Bananas taste great combined with lots of other fruits as well as vegetables, grains, and even some meat. Use ripe bananas for this puree, as they're easier to mash. Bananas tend to turn brown once peeled, so if you're not planning to use a whole banana, only peel the portion you're using and store the rest in the fridge. A ripe banana makes a great portable baby food when you're travelling.

I medium ripe banana, peeled

Place the banana in a bowl and mash with the back of a fork or spoon until smooth. Add a small amount of water, breast milk, or formula as needed to reach desired consistency. Alternatively, puree with a food processor or blender until smooth. Serve or store.

Banana puree can be stored in the refrigerator in an airtight container for 1 day or in the freezer for 3 months. Some discoloration and browning will occur with storage. If freezing, spoon individual portions into ice cube trays or baby food containers, then cover and freeze.

Flavor boost: cinnamon, cardamom, vanilla

Avocado Mash

Makes about ¾ cup

With nearly 20 vitamins and minerals in every serving, avocados are nutritional rock stars! Rich in heart-healthy monounsaturated fats, they have a buttery texture that adds creaminess to other purees like meat, seafood, beans, and grains. Use ripe avocados as they're easier to mash. Similar to banana, avocado also turns brown once it's peeled so if you're not planning to use a whole one, only use half and store the other half in the fridge (keep the pit in as it will help slow any browning). Once your baby is older and you've introduced them to lemon, you can also rub a little lemon juice on the avocado to prevent it from turning brown.

I medium ripe avocado

Cut the avocado in half lengthwise around the pit and twist to open. Wrap the half with the pit clinging to it in plastic wrap and reserve in the fridge for another serving. Scoop out the flesh from the remaining avocado half with a spoon. Place it in a bowl and mash with the back of a fork or spoon until smooth. Add a small amount of water, breast milk, or formula as needed to reach desired consistency. Alternatively, puree the avocado with a food processor or blender until smooth Serve or store.

Avocado puree can be stored in the refrigerator in an airtight container for 1 day. Avocado puree does not freeze well.

Flavor boost: cilantro, cumin, garlic

Baby's First Oatmeal
Cereal, page 87

Cereals

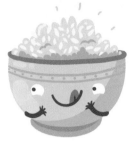

WHILE YOU'LL FIND THAT rice and other grains will soon be a staple in your baby's diet, how you prepare these grains depends on your baby's age and developmental stage. When you first introduce rice and other grains like barley and oats, it will be in the form of cereal. Although you can buy commercially prepared cereal, it's easy to make at home, which allows you to use only the most nutritious ingredients. Simply grind up the grain in a food processor, blender or spice grinder. Then, cook it on the stove like porridge. The cereal powder can be kept in the fridge in an airtight container so it makes sense to grind up a large batch of cereal and then cook up small portions as needed.

As your baby gets older and becomes more advanced developmentally, you can stop making cereal and cook the grains whole. Depending on their chewing ability, you can puree the grains a little after they're cooked or just leave them whole. Once your baby gets into finger foods, they'll have fun trying to pick up the grains and feed themselves.

Below are recipes for three of the most common cereals—rice, barley, and oats. The next chapter will include recipes on how to prepare these grains (along with some others) for older babies.

Keep in mind that commercially prepared cereal from the grocery store is fortified with iron (it usually provides 45 percent of your baby's daily iron needs). For this reason, it's often recommended as an important staple to keep in your pantry. If you're intending to make your own cereal, you'll need to discuss your baby's iron needs with your pediatrician. Babies can get iron from a variety of other sources, including breast milk, formula, meat, legumes (like lentils and beans), wheat germ, and dried fruit.

Baby's First Rice Cereal

Makes I cup

Rice cereal has traditionally been the most common first food recommended by doctors, although these recommendations are now changing. If you do give your baby rice cereal, consider making it yourself. You can use brown rice, a whole grain that's packed with important nutrients for your baby like manganese, selenium, B vitamins, and fiber. Look for short grain brown rice, as it will cook up softer and more tender than medium or long grain. Rice cereal tastes good mixed with a wide variety of fruit, vegetable, and meat purees and can also be used to thicken purees.

¼ cup brown rice, preferably short grain
I cup water

Puree the rice in a food processor or blender until it is a fine powder.

Place the water in a small saucepan and bring to a boil. Add the brown rice powder and reduce heat to low. Cook, whisking frequently, until the water is completely absorbed and the cereal is smooth, 5–7 minutes. Cool and serve or store. You can add breast milk, formula or water to thin the cereal to desired consistency.

Rice cereal powder can be kept in the fridge in an airtight container and then cooked as needed. You can also store cooked rice cereal in the refrigerator in an airtight container for 3 days or in the freezer for 3 months. If freezing, spoon individual portions into ice cube trays or baby food containers, then cover and freeze.

Baby's First Barley Cereal

Makes 1 cup

Barley is a nutritious whole grain with a slightly sweet, earthy flavor. It's a good first cereal because—like rice—it's non-allergenic and easy to digest. It's also rich in fiber, iron, selenium, and plenty of other nutrients. Barley cereal tastes good mixed with a wide variety of fruit, vegetable, and meat purees and can also be used to thicken purees.

¼ cup pearl barley
1 cup water

Puree the barley in a food processor or blender until it is a fine powder. Place the water in a small saucepan and bring to a boil. Add the barley powder, and reduce heat to low. Cook, whisking frequently, until the water is completely absorbed and the cereal is smooth, about 5 minutes. Cool and serve or store. You can add breast milk, formula, or water to thin the cereal to desired consistency. Cool before serving.

Barley cereal powder can be kept in the fridge in an airtight container and then cooked as needed. You can also store cooked barley cereal in the refrigerator in an airtight container for 3 days or in the freezer for 3 months. If freezing, spoon individual portions into ice cube trays or baby food containers, then cover and freeze.

Baby's First Oatmeal Cereal

Makes 1 cup

Oatmeal is an excellent starter cereal for babies, and you don't have to limit it to just breakfast. High in protein, fiber, and several vitamins and minerals, this whole grain has a flavor that many babies enjoy and it's less constipating than rice cereal. Oatmeal cereal tastes good mixed with a wide variety of fruit, vegetable, and meat purees and can also be used to thicken purees.

¼ cup old-fashioned or steel cut oats
1 cup water

Puree the oats in a food processor or blender until it is a fine powder. Place the water in a small saucepan and bring to a boil. Add the ground oats, and reduce heat to low. Cook, whisking frequently, until the water is completely absorbed and the cereal is smooth, about 5 minutes. Cool and serve or store. You can add breast milk, formula, or water to thin the cereal to desired consistency.

Oatmeal cereal powder can be stored in the fridge in an airtight container and then cooked as needed. You can also store cooked oatmeal cereal in the refrigerator in an airtight container for 3 days or in the freezer for 3 months. If freezing, spoon individual portions into ice cube trays or baby food containers, then cover and freeze.

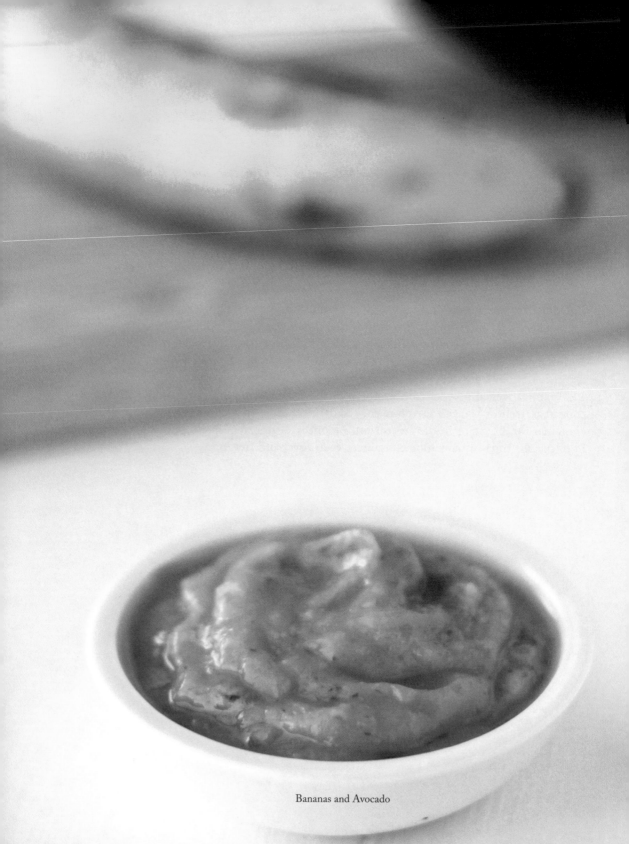

Bananas and Avocado

Tasty Combinations

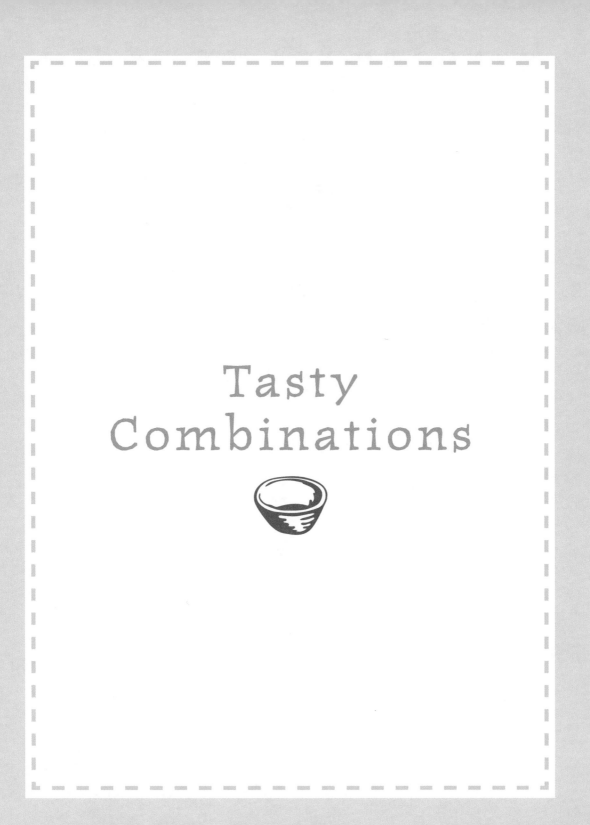

Once you've introduced individual purees to your baby, you can start combining purees to make tasty combinations. Below are a few of my favorite combinations, all using recipes from this chapter.

As your baby gets older, you can start incorporating a wider variety of foods in your combinations, including other fruits and vegetables, meat, legumes, grains, and yogurt.

- Cereal (rice, barley, or oatmeal) with any fruit puree
- Cereal (rice, barley, or oatmeal) with any vegetable puree
- Sweet potatoes and pears
- Sweet potatoes and bananas
- Sweet potatoes and butternut squash
- Butternut squash and apples
- Peas and carrots
- Peas and pears
- Carrots, apples, and parsnips
- Parsnips and pears
- Zucchini and apples
- Zucchini and potatoes
- Potatoes and peas
- Apples and avocado
- Apples and pears
- Bananas and pears
- Bananas and avocado
- Avocado, peas, and pears

FUN FLAVORS: 6–8 MONTHS

A T 6–8 MONTHS, YOUR goal for your baby should be to introduce them to a wide variety of nutritious ingredients and flavors. You are expanding your baby's palate and teaching them how to enjoy the natural flavors in these healthful, whole foods. You can introduce lots of different fruits, vegetables, grains, and meat, but hold off on giving cow's milk until 1 year (yogurt and some cheeses are fine to give after 6 months, as they're easier to digest).

There are a lot of purees in this section. Let your creative side run wild and make combinations of your own—just make sure you continue to follow the 3–5 day rule, and only introduce your baby to one new ingredient at a time. As your baby gets used to eating solids, you can start seasoning his or her food with some herbs and spices to make it tastier. You can also start adding a small amount of butter or oil for flavor and mouth feel; however, you shouldn't add any sugar or salt to your baby's food. If you feel like a dish needs some sweetness, add some fresh fruit puree instead.

When your baby first started solid foods, your purees should have been smooth and runny. As they get older and become more accustomed to solids, start making the purees thicker and lumpier. Many of the recipes in this section say to blend or puree to desired consistency. This is because you can adapt these recipes as your baby grows, adjusting the consistency based on their chewing ability.

There are several fruit purees in this chapter; for most of them, steaming instructions are given. Some fruits that are firm, like apples, are always going to need to be cooked in order to soften them enough to puree. But for other, softer fruits, like peaches and plums, the steaming step is optional depending on how ripe the fruit is and what stage your baby is at. When you first introduce fruits to babies—especially if you are introducing them at an early age—many pediatric sources recommend cooking them, because it makes them easier to digest. (Bananas and avocados are exceptions and never need to be cooked.)

As your baby gets a little older, you can skip the steaming step, especially if you're using soft, ripe fruit. As her or his tummy matures, your baby will be able to handle the fiber and sugars in raw fruit better than a younger baby who's just starting on solids. The fruit puree recipes in this chapter that have an optional steaming step are designated as "no-cook purees."

Many parents have questions about how much their baby should be eating. The answer is that it's highly variable—every baby progresses at a different pace. In terms of serving size, try starting out with about 2 tablespoons of solid food at a meal. Over the next several weeks, as your baby starts to eat more, increase it until they're eating about ¼ cup servings. Also, over the next several weeks (when your baby is ready), you should work up to three solid meals a day.

Don't worry if your baby doesn't eat a consistent amount at every meal. Remember, at this age you are just trying to get them used to the process of eating solid foods. Breast milk or formula is still your baby's primary source of nutrition at this point. If your baby doesn't seem too excited about a particular puree, don't give up; try it again later. You can also try mixing it with a puree that they do enjoy. Remember, babies often need multiple exposures to a food before they will accept them.

At this age, you can also introduce a sippy cup. You can give your little one a small amount of water, breast milk, or formula at meals to get them used to drinking from a cup.

The following is a sample menu for a 6–8 month old baby. Remember that all babies are unique and that this is just a general guideline. The amount and types of food that babies eat at each meal is highly variable. The most important thing is to follow your baby's individual needs and cues.

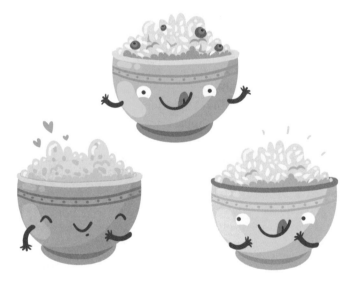

SAMPLE MENU FOR A 6- TO 8-MONTH-OLD

MEAL	SAMPLE MENU	EXAMPLES USING RECIPES FROM THIS BOOK
Breakfast	· 2–4 tablespoons cereal or grains · 2–4 tablespoons fruit or· vegetable · 4–6 ounces breast milk or iron-fortified formula	· Baby's First Oatmeal Cereal (page 87) with Blueberry Puree (page 106) · Baby's First Oatmeal Cereal (page 87) with Apple Strawberry Compote (page 130) · Baby's First Rice Cereal (page 85) with Peach Puree (page 102) · Apricots, Bananas, and Barley (page 127)
Mid-Morning	· 4–6 ounces breast milk or iron-fortified formula	
Lunch	· 2–4 tablespoons cereal or grains · 2–4 tablespoons fruit or vegetable · 4–6 ounces breast milk or iron-fortified formula	· Baby's First Rice Cereal (page 85) with Gingery Carrots and Apples (page 127) · Baby's First Barley Cereal (page 86) with Cauliflower Puree (page 97) · Butternut Squash Risotto (page 128) · Baby's First Rice Cereal (page 85) with Broccoli, Peas, and Pear (page 129) · Tropical Rice Pudding (page 131)
Mid-Afternoon	· 4–6 ounces breast milk or iron-fortified formula or ½ serving dairy or 2–4 tablespoons fruit or vegetable	· Green Bean Puree (page 96) · Apricot Puree (page 104) · Cherries, Berries, and Yogurt (page 126) · Purple Power (page 132)
Dinner	· 1–3 tablespoons protein* · 2–4 tablespoons vegetable or fruit · 2–4 tablespoons cereal or grains · 4–6 ounces breast milk or iron-fortified formula	· Baby's Chicken Puree and Parsnips (page 112) with Baby's First Rice Cereal (page 85) · Baby's Beef Puree and Butternut Squash (page 114) with Baby's First Barley Cereal (page 86) · Turkey and Taters (page 113) with Baby's First Rice Cereal (page 85) · Baby's Fish Dinner (page 116) with Baby's First Oatmeal Cereal (page 87) · Black Beans, Mango, and Avocado (page 122) with Baby's First Rice Cereal (page 85)
Before Bed	· 6–8 ounces breast milk or iron-fortified formula	

Protein includes meat, poultry, fish, cooked legumes (like beans and lentils), tofu, and eggs

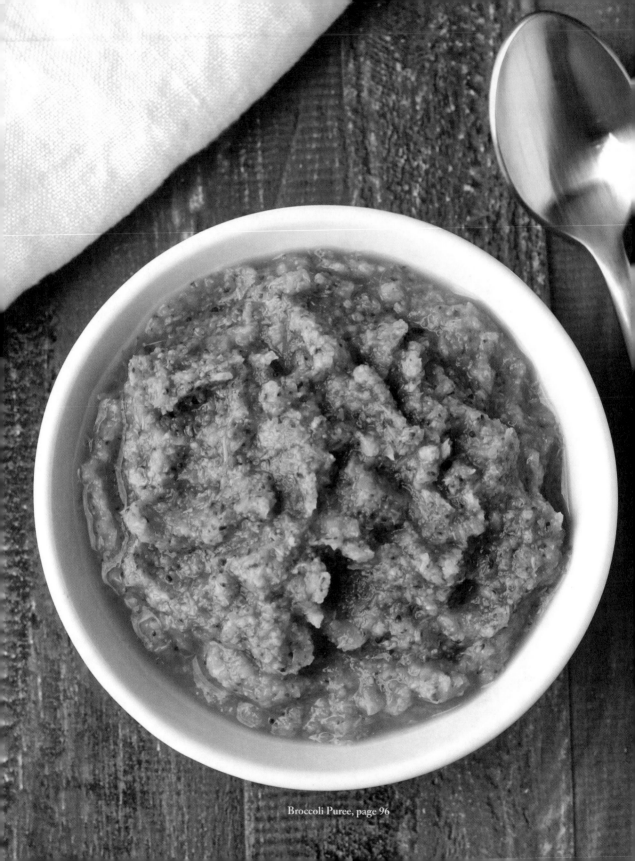

Broccoli Puree, page 96

Vibrant
Vegetables

Green Bean Puree

Makes 2 cups

Green beans are a rich source of dietary fiber, Vitamin A, Vitamin C, Vitamin K, folate, and manganese. They can be very fibrous, so use a blender to get a smoother puree. Otherwise, after pureeing, you can pass the puree through a strainer. Frozen green beans tend to give a smoother puree than do fresh green beans, so you may want to consider making a trip to the freezer section. Green bean puree is delicious alone or mixed with sweet vegetables (like sweet potatoes or carrots), yogurt, or rice.

I pound green beans, washed thoroughly

Snap or cut the ends off the beans. Set the beans in a steamer basket over boiling water. Cover and steam until tender, 7–8 minutes (10 minutes if using frozen).

Puree with a food processor or blender until smooth. Add a small amount of fresh water as needed to reach desired consistency. If needed, pass the puree through a strainer to get rid of any fibrous material. Cool and serve or store.

Green bean puree can be stored in the refrigerator in an airtight container for 3 days or in the freezer for 3 months. If freezing, spoon individual portions into ice cube trays or baby food containers, then cover and freeze.

Flavor boost: basil, dill, marjoram

Broccoli Puree

Makes about 1½ cups

Broccoli is a nutritional powerhouse, rich in antioxidants, fiber and several vitamins and minerals including Vitamin C, Vitamin K, folate and potassium. Broccoli is best steamed, as boiling it causes it to lose significant amounts of Vitamin C. For a creamier puree, mix broccoli with potato, sweet potato, or carrot puree. If your baby doesn't like the strong taste of broccoli, you can try mixing it with sweet-tasting vegetables or fruits like sweet potato, pumpkin, butternut squash, apple, or pear.

4 cups broccoli florets

Place the broccoli in a steamer basket set over boiling water. Cover and steam until tender, about 8–10 minutes. Remove broccoli from the steamer, reserving cooking liquid.

Puree with a food processor or blender until smooth. Add a small amount of the cooking liquid as needed to reach desired consistency. Cool and serve or store.

Broccoli puree can be stored in the refrigerator in an airtight container for 3 days or in the freezer for 3 months. If freezing, spoon individual portions into ice cube trays or baby food containers, then cover and freeze.

Flavor boost: garlic, ginger, oregano

Cauliflower Puree

Makes about 1½ cups

Cauliflower is a cruciferous vegetable that's packed with powerful antioxidants as well as an impressive array of nutrients including protein, fiber, Vitamin C, Vitamin K, folate, and choline. Cauliflower has a neutral flavor and pairs well with a wide variety of fruits, vegetables, grains, and legumes including apple, pear, broccoli, rice, lentils, and chickpeas.

4 cups cauliflower florets

Place the cauliflower in a steamer basket set over boiling water. Cover and steam until tender, 12–15 minutes. Remove cauliflower from the steamer, reserving the cooking liquid.

Puree in a food processor or blender until smooth. Add a small amount of the cooking liquid as needed to reach desired consistency. Cool and serve or store.

Cauliflower puree can be stored in the refrigerator in an airtight container for 3 days or in the freezer for 3 months. If freezing, spoon individual portions into ice cube trays or baby food containers, then cover and freeze.

Flavor boost: curry powder, paprika, turmeric

Spinach Puree

Makes 1¼ cups

Spinach is a true superfood, packed with a wide variety of essential vitamins and minerals. You can use fresh or frozen spinach to make this puree. If using frozen spinach, defrost it according to package directions and proceed with the rest of the recipe. Spinach is one of the vegetables with the highest pesticide residues so try to buy organic when possible. For a creamier puree, mix spinach with potato, sweet potato, butternut squash, or carrot puree.

1 container (10 ounces) fresh spinach, stems removed

Wash the spinach thoroughly. Place the spinach in a steamer basket set over boiling water. Cover and steam until tender, about 5 minutes. Remove spinach from the steamer.

Puree spinach in a food processor or blender until smooth. Add a small amount of fresh water as needed to reach desired consistency. Cool and serve or store.

Kale Puree: Use kale instead of spinach

Flavor boost: coriander, garlic, nutmeg

Spinach and Sweet Potatoes

Makes 1 cup

Sweet potatoes add creaminess and sweetness to spinach puree. You can also substitute potatoes, butternut squash, or carrots for the sweet potato.

½ cup Spinach Puree (above)
½ cup Sweet Potato Puree (page 68)

Mix all ingredients together in a bowl. Serve or store.

Beet Puree

Makes about 2 cups

Beets are rich in several nutrients including fiber, folate, Vitamin C, potassium, and manganese. Red beets are the most common type sold in stores but they also come in different varieties, like golden and Chioggia (striped). Beets tend to stain so be careful when preparing and serving them; you may want to wear gloves. The beet greens are very nutritious as well so save them and use them in a salad for yourself.

3 beets (about 12 ounces)

Preheat oven to 400°F.

Remove the beet greens and trim the stems, leaving an inch of the stems and the root intact. Wash the beets thoroughly.

Wrap each beat in foil and place them on a baking sheet. Roast in the oven until tender, 50–60 minutes. Remove from oven and cool slightly.

Trim off the beet roots and rub the skin off. Chop the beets and place them in a food processor. Puree until smooth, adding water 1 tablespoon at a time, to reach desired consistency.

You can also steam beets if you're short on time. Thoroughly wash and peel the raw beets. Chop them and place the pieces in a steamer basket set over boiling water. Cover and steam until tender, about 12–15 minutes. Puree as above, using fresh water.

Flavor boost: chives, dill, mint

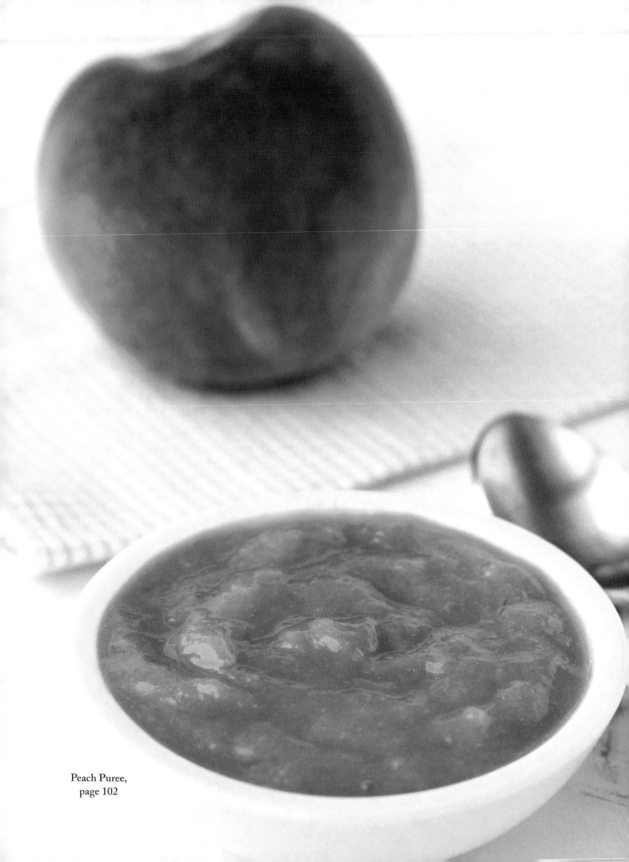

Peach Puree,
page 102

Fantastic
Fruits

Peach Puree

Makes 1½ cups

Peaches are packed with Vitamin C and Vitamin A as well as fiber and potassium. Peach puree can be mixed with a wide variety of other purees to add a bright, sweet flavor. Try combining peaches with iron-rich purees like meats, as the Vitamin C will help your baby absorb the iron. Peaches are often on the list of the most heavily contaminated fruits and vegetables so try to buy organic when possible.

4 peaches, washed, peeled, and pitted

Chop the peaches and place them in a steamer basket set over boiling water. Cover and steam until tender, 4–6 minutes.

Puree with an immersion blender or food processor until smooth. Cool and serve or store.

Peach puree can be stored in the refrigerator in an airtight container for 3 days or in the freezer for 3 months. If freezing, spoon individual portions into ice cube trays or baby food containers, then cover and freeze.

Nectarine Puree: Use nectarines instead of peaches.

No-Cook Puree: If peaches are ripe and soft, then you can puree without steaming.

Flavor boost: cinnamon, ginger, nutmeg, vanilla

When peeling peaches (as well as nectarines, plums, apricots, and tomatoes), you can peel them with a vegetable peeler. An alternative way of peeling them is to blanch them in boiling water first—the peel will then come off easily. To do this, score the bottom of the peaches with an "x" and plunge them in boiling water for 1 minute. Remove the peaches with a slotted spoon and plunge them into a bowl of ice water. After about 1 minute, or when cool enough to handle, slip off the skin with your fingers or a small knife.

Plum Puree

Makes 1 cup

Plums have a mild flavor and complement many other fruits and vegetables. Plums are a very good source of Vitamin C and also have a good amount of Vitamin A, Vitamin K, and fiber. See page 108 for dried plum (prune) puree.

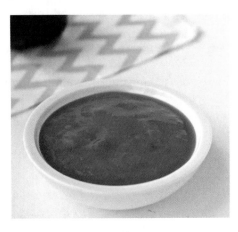

4 plums, washed, peeled and pitted

Chop the plums and place them in a steamer basket set over boiling water. Cover and steam until tender, 5–7 minutes.

Puree with an immersion blender or food processor until smooth. Cool and serve or store.

Plum puree can be stored in the refrigerator in an airtight container for 3 days or in the freezer for 3 months. If freezing, spoon individual portions into ice cube trays or baby food containers, then cover and freeze.

No-Cook Puree: If plums are ripe and soft, then you can puree without steaming.

Flavor boost: allspice, cinnamon, cloves, vanilla

Cherry Puree

Makes about 1 cup

Packed as they are with antioxidants, cherries are undeniable nutritional powerhouses. To remove the pits, use a cherry or olive pitter, or cut around the pit with a small knife.

Cherries have only a short season in the summer, so for the rest of the year, buy frozen (they're convenient, easy, and affordable). Plus, you won't have to spend time pitting them.

2 dozen fresh or frozen cherries, washed and pitted

Place the cherries in a steamer basket set over boiling water. Cover and steam until tender, about 3 minutes.

Puree with an immersion blender or food processor until smooth. Cool and serve or store.

Cherry puree can be stored in the refrigerator in an airtight container for 3 days or in the freezer for 3 months. If freezing, spoon individual portions into ice cube trays or baby food containers, then cover and freeze.

No-Cook Puree: If cherries are ripe and soft, then you can puree without steaming.

Flavor boost: cinnamon, lime juice, mint

Apricot Puree

Makes about 1 cup

Fresh apricots are one of the first signs of summer. They have a very short season so when you see them at the market, be sure to snatch them up! Apricots are lovely, golden-colored fruit with velvety flesh and a sweet, slightly tart flavor. They are packed with powerful antioxidants and also provide plenty of Vitamin A, Vitamin C, and fiber. When they're out of season, you can use dried apricots (see page 109).

4 apricots, washed

Cut the apricots in half and remove the pits. Place the apricots halves in a steamer basket set over boiling water. Cover and steam until tender, 4–6 minutes. Remove the skins.

Puree with an immersion blender or food processor until smooth. Cool and serve or store.

Apricot puree can be stored in the refrigerator in an airtight container for 3 days or in the freezer for 3 months. If freezing, spoon individual portions into ice cube trays or baby food containers, then cover and freeze.

No-Cook Puree: If apricots are ripe and soft, then you can puree without steaming.

Flavor boost: cardamom, ginger, vanilla

Note: You can also blanch the apricots in boiling water to remove the skins (see page 102).

Papaya Puree

Makes about 1 cup

Papayas are rich in beta-carotene, which gets converted to Vitamin A in the body. They're also packed with Vitamin C, so try combining this puree with iron-rich foods (like chicken or pork) for better absorption. Because papayas are rich in fiber, they can help if your baby is constipated. Papaya contains papain, an enzyme that breaks down protein and aids in digestion. It is for this reason that you can find it in many meat tenderizers.

1 medium papaya, washed and peeled

Cut the papaya in half lengthwise and remove the black seeds. Chop the flesh and place it in a steamer basket set over boiling water. Cover and steam until tender, 7–8 minutes.

Puree with an immersion blender or food processor until smooth. Cool and serve or store.

Papaya puree can be stored in the refrigerator in an airtight container for 3 days or in the freezer for 3 months. If freezing, spoon individual portions into ice cube trays or baby food containers, then cover and freeze.

No-Cook Puree: If papaya is ripe and soft, then you can puree without steaming.

Flavor boost: ginger, mint, lime juice

Mango Puree

Makes about 1 cup

Babies love the sweet flavor of mango, a nutrient-dense fruit that's loaded with antioxidants. This puree is also rich in vitamins and minerals including Vitamin A, Vitamin C, and Vitamin B6, to boost your baby's immune system and help prevent chronic diseases. Mangoes are also a rich source of fiber.

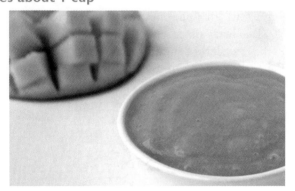

1 medium mango, washed and peeled

Slice down the sides of the mango on either side of the pit. Chop the flesh and place it in a steamer basket set over boiling water. Cover and steam until tender, 3–5 minutes.

Puree with an immersion blender or food processor until smooth. Cool and serve or store.

Mango puree can be stored in the refrigerator in an airtight container for 3 days or in the freezer for 3 months. If freezing, spoon individual portions into ice cube trays or baby food containers, then cover and freeze.

No-Cook Puree: If mango is ripe and soft, then you can puree without steaming.

Flavor boost: ginger, mint, lime juice

Blueberry Puree

Makes 1½ cups

Valued for their high level of antioxidants, blueberries are also rich in Vitamin C, Vitamin K, manganese, and fiber. Also, they are less allergenic than other berries. You can use frozen blueberries when they're out of season. Frozen berries are convenient, economical, and last a long time (as opposed to fresh berries, which spoil quickly).

1 pint (2 cups) blueberries, washed

Place the blueberries in a steamer basket set over boiling water. Cover and steam until tender, about 3 minutes.

Puree with an immersion blender or food processor until smooth. If desired, strain the puree through a fine-mesh sieve to remove the skins. Cool and serve or store.

Blueberry puree can be stored in the refrigerator in an airtight container for 3 days or in the freezer for 3 months. If freezing, spoon individual portions into ice cube trays or baby food containers, then cover and freeze.

No-Cook Puree: If blueberries are ripe, you can skip the steaming step.

Flavor boost: Cinnamon, nutmeg, thyme

Blueberry Banana Puree

Makes ⅓ cup

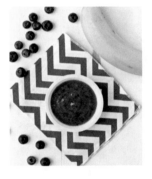

This lovely lavender puree was my daughter Sienna's favorite when she was a baby. It's rich in potassium, fiber, Vitamin C, and Vitamin K. You can stir in some Greek yogurt for a boost of protein and calcium.

1 banana, peeled
3 tablespoons blueberry puree (page 106)

Mash the banana and blueberry puree together in a bowl until smooth. Alternatively, you puree them in a food processor or blender until smooth. Serve or store.

Strawberry Puree

Makes 1 cup

Strawberries are very nutritious, containing high amounts of Vitamin C, fiber, manganese and antioxidants. However, they also have some of the highest amounts of pesticide residue. Buy organic when possible; you can use frozen out of season. Because strawberries can be allergenic, old recommendations were to delay introducing them to children until 1 year of age. Current recommendations give them the green light after 6 months. However, if you have a family history of allergies, talk to your pediatrician before introducing them to your baby.

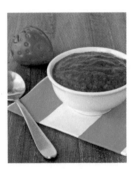

1 pint (2 cups) strawberries, washed

Place the strawberries in a steamer basket set over boiling water. Cover and steam until tender, about 3 minutes.

Puree with an immersion blender or food processor until smooth. If desired, strain the puree through a fine-mesh sieve to remove the seeds. Cool and serve or store.

Strawberry puree can be stored in the refrigerator in an airtight container for 3 days or in the freezer for 3 months. If freezing, spoon individual portions into ice cube trays or baby food containers, then cover and freeze.

Raspberry or Blackberry Puree: Use raspberries or blackberries instead of strawberries

No-Cook Puree: If strawberries are ripe, you can skip the steaming step.

Flavor boost: Basil, lemon juice, mint, vanilla

Pretty in Pink Raspberry Pear Puree

Makes 1½ cups

Sweet pears nicely balance out the tart raspberries in this lovely pink puree. Serve it plain or stir it into oatmeal or other cereals.

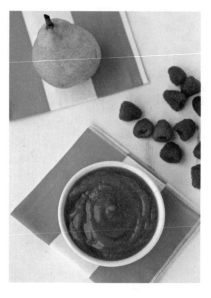

2 ripe pears, peeled and chopped
1 cup raspberries

Puree the pears and raspberries with a food processor or blender until smooth. If desired, strain the puree through a fine-mesh sieve to remove the seeds. Serve or store.

Dried Plum (Prune) Puree

Makes 1 cup

Dried fruit is one of the only instances when I recommend boiling, as you will need to rehydrate the fruit. Use this recipe to make dried plum (prune) puree or dried apricot puree. Both are rich in fiber, which helps to maintain bowel integrity and alleviate constipation. They are also a good source of iron and potassium, which become more concentrated in the drying process.

1 cup pitted dried plums (prunes)

Place the dried plums in a saucepan with 1 cup water and bring to a boil. Reduce to a simmer and cook until soft, 8–10 minutes.

Transfer the plums to a food processor, reserving the cooking liquid. Puree until smooth, adding the cooking liquid, a small amount at a time, as needed to achieve desired consistency.

Dried plum puree can be stored in the refrigerator in an airtight container for 3 days or in the freezer for 3 months. If freezing, spoon individual portions into ice cube trays or baby food containers, then cover and freeze. Dried fruit purees won't freeze completely solid but will be slightly soft or tacky.

Dried Apricot Puree: Substitute dried apricots for dried plums

Flavor boost: cinnamon, cloves, vanilla

Melon Puree

Makes about 1 cup

This recipe can be used for cantaloupe, honeydew, or other melons. Cantaloupe is the most nutrient-rich melon. High in water content, cantaloupe doesn't freeze well, so it's better to make small batches and use the rest of the melon for another purpose (like a fruit salad for yourself). You can freeze chunks or slices of melon to use when your baby is teething, as the cold will be soothing. Soft pieces of melon also make for good finger food.

1 small cantaloupe or honeydew, washed

Cut the melon in half and scoop out the seeds. Remove the rind from half of the melon and chop into chunks. Reserve the remaining melon half for another use.

Puree with an immersion blender or food processor until smooth. Serve or store.

Melon puree can be stored in the refrigerator in an airtight container for 3 days. Melon puree does not freeze well.

Flavor boost: lemon juice, mint

Baby's Chicken
Puree, page 112

Mighty Meat
and Fish

Baby's Chicken Puree

Makes about 2 cups

Meat purees are an excellent way to boost your baby's iron intake. Chicken is a good first meat for babies; it has a mild flavor and is easily digested. You can make chicken puree for your baby by roasting or poaching chicken breasts or thighs and then pureeing them, but I prefer to start with ground chicken, which gives a smoother puree. Whenever possible, choose organic, free-range chicken, which is not treated with any antibiotics, steroids, or hormones.

I pound ground chicken

Heat a large skillet over medium high heat and add the chicken. Brown the chicken, breaking it up with a spatula or wooden spoon, until cooked, 6–8 minutes. Add a small amount of water to the skillet as needed to prevent the meat from sticking. Cool slightly.

Transfer the chicken to a food processor or blender using a slotted spoon. Puree to desired consistency, adding a small amount of water as needed to achieve desired consistency.

Chicken puree can be stored in the refrigerator in an airtight container for 3 days or in the freezer for 3 months. If freezing, spoon individual portions into ice cube trays or baby food containers, then cover and freeze.

Baby's Turkey Puree: Use ground turkey instead of chicken

Flavor boost: sage, tarragon, thyme, rosemary

Mixing chicken puree together with fruits, vegetables, and grains may make it more enjoyable for your baby and in turn, more likely for them to eat it. Mixing chicken with Vitamin C–rich foods like mango, apricot, peaches, papaya, and broccoli will help them to better absorb the iron in the chicken.

Here are some good combinations with chicken:

Chicken and Fruit variation (makes ¼ cup): Stir together 2 tablespoons Baby's Chicken Puree and 2 tablespoons Mango Puree (page 105), Apricot Puree (page 104), Pear Puree (page 77), Peach Puree (page 102) or Papaya Puree (page 105).

Chicken and Vegetable variation (makes ¼ cup): Stir together 2 tablespoons Baby's Chicken Puree and 2 tablespoons Parsnip Puree (page 72), Green Bean Puree (page 96), Broccoli Puree (page 96), Potato Puree (page 73) or Butternut Squash Puree (page 69).

Chicken and Grain variation (makes ¼ cup): Stir together 2 tablespoons Baby's Chicken Puree and 2 tablespoons Baby's First Rice Cereal (page 85) or Baby's First Barley Cereal (page 86).

Did You Know?

Although chicken breasts are the most commonly purchased cut of chicken, you should try to give your baby dark meat in addition to white meat. Dark meat cuts, like thighs and legs, actually have more iron and zinc than white meat. Dark meat also has more fat, which can make it easier to puree to a smooth consistency. Remember, babies need fat for their growth and development!

Turkey and Taters

Makes I cup

With its mild flavor, turkey is an excellent choice of meat for babies. It's also a rich source of protein, iron, and zinc. Turkey and potatoes are a classic combination. Plus the vitamin C in the potatoes will help your baby better absorb the iron in the turkey. This is a nice dish to serve your baby at the holiday table.

- ½ cup Baby's Turkey Puree (page 112)
- ½ cup Sweet Potato Puree (page 68) or Potato Puree (page 73)
- ⅛ teaspoon dried sage or thyme (optional)

Mix all ingredients together in a bowl. Serve or store.

Green Turkey and Taters variation: Stir in ½ cup Green Bean Puree, Sweet Pea Puree, or Broccoli Puree into the Turkey and Taters.

Baby's Beef Puree

Makes about 2 cups

Beef is an excellent source of protein, iron, zinc, and B vitamins, which are crucial for your baby's development. Whenever possible, choose organic beef, which is not treated with any antibiotics, steroids, or hormones.

I pound ground beef

Heat a large skillet over medium high heat and add the beef. Brown the beef, breaking it up with a spatula or wooden spoon, until cooked, 7–8 minutes. Add a small amount of water to the skillet as needed to prevent the meat from sticking. Drain the fat and cool slightly.

Remove beef from the skillet using a slotted spoon, leaving the fat behind. Transfer beef to a food processor or blender. Puree to desired consistency, adding a small amount of water as needed to achieve desired consistency.

Beef puree can be stored in the refrigerator in an airtight container for 3 days or in the freezer for 3 months. If freezing, spoon individual portions into ice cube trays or baby food containers, then cover and freeze.

Baby's Lamb Puree: use ground lamb instead of beef.

Flavor boost: cumin, garlic, thyme, rosemary

Beef and Fruit variation (makes ¼ cup): Stir together 2 tablespoons Baby's Beef Puree and 2 tablespoons Mango Puree (page 105) or Apricot Puree (page 104).

Beef and Vegetable variation (makes ¼ cup): Stir together 2 tablespoons Baby's Beef Puree and 2 tablespoons Potato Puree (page 73), Sweet Potato Puree (page 68), Carrot Puree (page 72), Green Bean Puree (page 96), Broccoli Puree (page 96), Sweet Pea Puree (page 70) or Butternut Squash Puree (page 69).

Beef and Grain variation (makes ¼ cup): Stir together 2 tablespoons Baby's Beef Puree and 2 tablespoons Baby's First Rice Cereal (page 85) or Baby's First Barley Cereal (page 86).

Super Salmon Puree

Makes about 1 cup

Salmon is a true superfood! It's packed with nutrients, including omega-3 fatty acids, which are crucial for your baby's brain and eye development. Try to use wild salmon if possible. Alaskan salmon in particular is low in mercury, is environmentally friendly, and often has a superior flavor. If it's too expensive, choose a sustainably farmed salmon.

Water or low-sodium chicken or vegetable broth
8 ounces salmon filets, skinned

To Poach the Salmon:

Fill a large saucepan with about 2 inches of water or broth and bring to a simmer. Add the salmon to the pan in a single layer, making sure it is covered by liquid (add more liquid if needed).

Turn the heat to low so that the water is bubbling gently and cover the pan. Cook 7–10 minutes until salmon is cooked through. Drain the fish, reserving some of the cooking liquid.

To Roast the Salmon:

Preheat oven to 400°F.

Brush a baking sheet lightly with olive oil. Place the salmon on the baking sheet and cook in the oven for 15 minutes or until the flesh flakes easily with a fork. Remove from the oven and cool.

Once the Salmon is Cooked:

Break the salmon into pieces, checking for any small bones. Transfer the salmon to a food processor with a small amount of the cooking liquid and puree to desired consistency. Or, when the baby is older, mash the fish with a fork. Cool and serve or store.

Flavor boost: add a bay leaf, dill sprigs, or lemon slices to the poaching liquid

Salmon and Avocado Mash

Makes ½ cup

A combination of two superfoods, this puree will provide your baby with plenty of the nutrients that they need to grow big and strong! Avocado adds a nice creaminess to the salmon as well as a rich, buttery flavor.

¼ cup cooked, flaked salmon (see page 115)
¼ cup diced avocado

Using a potato masher or fork, mash salmon and avocado together in a bowl. If desired, puree the mixture in a food processor to desired consistency.

Baby's Fish Dinner

Makes about 2½ cups

Fish is a great source of lean protein and omega-3 fatty acids, as well as a host of other beneficial vitamins and minerals. Use a mild white (low mercury) fish like cod, flounder, or tilapia. You can make this dish with just fish and potatoes or you can combine it with any vegetable puree such as carrots or peas.

1 large russet potato, washed, peeled, and chopped
8 ounces flounder, cod, or other white fish fillet, cut into 6 pieces
¼ cup Carrot Puree (page 72) or Sweet Pea Puree (page 70)

Place the chopped potatoes in a steamer basket set over boiling water. Cover and steam 8 minutes. Add the fish and cook for 6–8 more minutes, or until the potatoes are tender and fish is cooked through. Remove the potatoes and fish from the steamer, reserving cooking liquid. Cool slightly.

Transfer the potatoes and fish to a food processor, along with the carrot or pea puree and 3–4 tablespoons of the cooking liquid. Puree to desired consistency, adding more liquid as needed.

Flavor boost: basil, dill, mint

Baby's Fish Dinner,
page 116

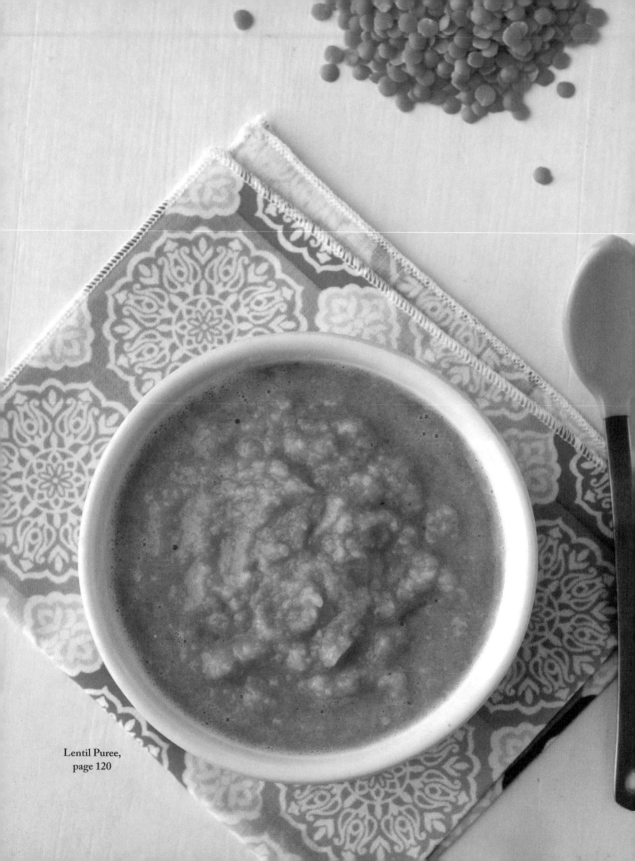

Lentil Puree,
page 120

Lovely Legumes

Lentil Puree

Makes 1 ½ cups

Lentils are rich in protein, iron, and antioxidants. They are an especially good choice for vegetarian babies as a source of protein. You can use any type of lentil in this recipe—red, brown, yellow, or green. I like to use red or yellow (moong dal) lentils for baby food because they cook quickly, puree to a smooth consistency, and may cause less gas than other varieties. Whatever type of lentils you choose, soak them first and then drain the soaking liquid, as it will get rid of many of the starches that cause digestive woes.

I cup lentils, rinsed

Bring a medium saucepan of water to a boil and add the lentils. Lower to a simmer and simmer until lentils are soft, about 20 minutes. Drain the water, reserving some of the cooking water.

Transfer the lentils to a food processor and puree until smooth, adding a small amount of the cooking liquid as needed. Cool and serve or store.

Flavor boost: cumin, curry powder, garlic

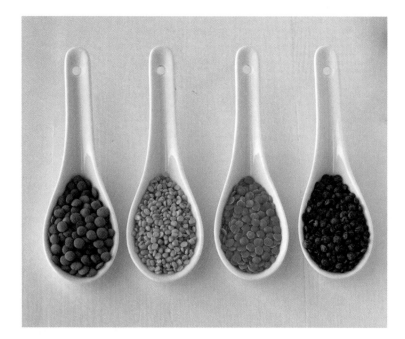

Red Lentil and Cauliflower Puree

Makes 1 cup

Red lentils have a mild flavor and can be mixed with a wide variety of vegetables, fruit and meat.

½ cup Lentil Puree using red lentils (see page 120)
½ cup Cauliflower Puree (see page 97)

In a medium bowl, combine the red lentil puree and cauliflower puree. Add water by the tablespoon as needed to thin puree to desired consistency. Serve or store.

Flavor boost: Parmesan cheese, ginger

Black Bean Puree

Makes about 1½ cups

Beans are a rich source of protein; they're also inexpensive. Dried beans take longer to cook, so if you're pressed for time, canned beans are a great convenience product. This recipe can also be used with pinto beans, kidney beans, cannellini beans, or other varieties. If you have leftovers, add some chicken or vegetable stock and make black bean soup for the rest of the family. This puree can also be used as a dip when your baby starts on finger foods (add some yogurt for creaminess).

¼ pound (about ½ cup) dried black beans or 1 can (15 ounces) low-sodium
black beans

If using dried beans, soak them overnight in a bowl of water. Drain and rinse. Place the beans in a large pot of water and bring to a boil. Reduce to a simmer and simmer until tender, 1–2 hours. Drain and rinse the cooked beans.

If using canned beans, drain and rinse the canned beans.

Transfer beans to a food processor and add a few tablespoons water or cooking liquid. Puree to desired consistency, adding more liquid as needed to thin the puree. Alternatively, you can also mash the beans with a fork or potato masher. Cool and serve or store.

Flavor boost: cumin, lime juice, chili powder

Black Beans, Mango, and Avocado

Makes 2 cups

Take your black beans up a notch with the addition of sweet mango and creamy avocado! Once your baby is old enough for finger foods, you can serve this dish without pureeing. It also makes an excellent salsa when served with grilled chicken, fish, or pork.

I can (15 ounces) low-sodium black beans, drained and rinsed
½ cup diced mango
½ cup diced avocado

Heat the beans and mango in a medium saucepan over medium heat with 2–4 tablespoons water. Cook on low heat until beans are heated through and mango is softened, 5–10 minutes. Add the avocado.

Mash the mixture with a fork or potato masher or transfer to a food processor and puree to desired consistency. Cool and serve or store.

Flavor boost: cumin, lime juice, cilantro

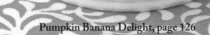
Pumpkin Banana Delight, page 126

Yellow Lentils and Rice
(Khichdi), page 129

More Tasty Combinations

Cherries, Berries, and Yogurt

Makes 1 cup

The combination of cherries and berries in this recipe makes for a delicious puree. It's even better when swirled into creamy yogurt, for a delightful treat that your baby will love! Yogurt is a good source of calcium, and if you use Greek yogurt, your baby will be getting an extra protein boost. (You can substitute any fruit puree in this recipe.)

¼ cup Cherry Puree (page 103)
¼ cup any Berry Puree (like blueberry, raspberry, or strawberry) (pages 106–108)
½ cup plain, whole milk yogurt

Mix all ingredients together in a bowl. Serve immediately, or cover and refrigerate.

Pumpkin Banana Delight

Makes ½ cup

Little ones will love this rich, creamy treat. When they get older, you can even spread it on crackers or toast or stir it into their oatmeal. Be sure to buy 100 percent pure canned pumpkin, not pumpkin pie filling, which has sugar and other ingredients added to it.

¼ cup fresh or canned pumpkin
    puree
1 medium banana, peeled and sliced
Pinch of cinnamon, cardamom, or
    ginger

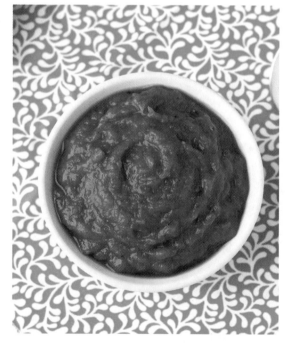

Puree the pumpkin, banana and cinnamon together in a food processor until smooth. Alternatively, mash the ingredients together in a bowl with a fork. Serve or store.

Gingery Carrots and Apples

Makes 1½ cups

This brightly colored puree is rich in vitamin A, vitamin C, potassium, and fiber. Ginger adds flavor and also aids in digestion. Serve it plain or stir in some Greek yogurt to add creaminess as well as a boost of protein and calcium.

4 carrots, peeled and chopped
1 apple, washed, peeled and chopped
⅛ teaspoon ground ginger

1 tablespoon plain, whole milk Greek yogurt (optional)

Place the carrots and apples in a steamer basket set over boiling water. Cover and steam until tender, 10–12 minutes. Cool slightly.

Transfer to a food processor or blender with the ginger. Puree until smooth, adding a small amount of water as needed to reach desired consistency.

To serve, place 2 tablespoons of the carrot apple mixture in a small bowl and stir in the Greek yogurt, if using. Store the remaining puree in the fridge or freezer.

This puree makes a nice base for carrot ginger soup. Double the recipe and add vegetable or chicken broth to the puree to make a delicious soup for the rest of the family. Season with salt and pepper, to taste.

Apricots, Bananas, and Barley

Makes ¾ cup

This delicious dish combines healthy whole grains with nutrient-rich apricots and banana. If you can't find fresh apricots, you can substitute dried.

¼ cup Baby's First Barley Cereal (page 86)
¼ cup Apricot Puree (page 104) or dried apricot puree (page 109)
¼ cup Banana Mash (page 80)

Mix all ingredients together in a small bowl. Serve immediately or cover and refrigerate.

Cantaloupe, Peaches, and Cottage Cheese

Makes 1 cup

Cottage cheese, a mixture of cheese curds and whey, is made by curdling cow's milk and then draining it without pressing it. Cottage cheese is a good source of calcium, healthy fats, and protein. It comes in small-curd and large-curd varieties, with small curds being easier for a baby to tolerate early on. Once they start exploring finger foods, you can try large curds and let them have fun picking the pieces up. Although cow's milk shouldn't be given before 1 year, cottage cheese is fine (much like other cheeses and yogurt). Cottage cheese tastes good with a wide variety of fruits, including blueberries, pineapple, pears, and apples.

½ cup whole milk cottage cheese
¼ cup Cantaloupe Puree (page 109)
¼ cup Peach Puree (page 102)

Mix all ingredients together in a small bowl. For a smoother consistency, puree in a food processor or blender.

This recipe can be stored in the refrigerator for up to 3 days, but does not freeze well.

Butternut Squash Risotto

Makes about 1½ cups

Risotto is an Italian rice dish, and is traditionally made by adding liquid in several increments. While this does result in a delicious finished product, it takes a while to make. You'll still get a nice creamy texture adding the broth all at once and you'll save a lot of time. You can make this recipe with pretty much any vegetable puree including sweet potato, zucchini, carrot, beet, or sweet pea. As your baby gets older, you can add soft cooked pieces of squash or other vegetables instead of purees.

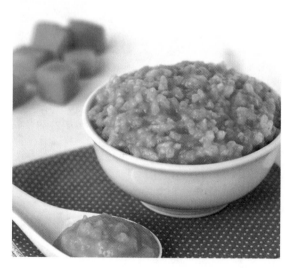

½ cup arborio rice
2 cups low-sodium chicken or vegetable broth or water
½ cup Butternut Squash Puree (page 69)

1 teaspoon unsalted butter
½ teaspoon chopped fresh sage or thyme (optional)

Bring the rice and broth to a boil in a medium saucepan. Reduce heat to low and cover. Simmer, stirring occasionally, until the liquid is absorbed and rice is creamy, 20–25 minutes. Remove from heat and let stand for 5–10 minutes.

Stir in the butternut squash puree, butter, and sage. Puree risotto to desired consistency using an immersion blender or food processor. Add a small amount of broth or water as needed to thin the puree.

Broccoli, Peas, and Pear

Makes 1½ cups

It's a good idea to introduce green vegetables into your baby's diet from an early age. Mixing stronger-flavored veggies like broccoli with milder, sweeter purees like pears and peas may help your little one accept them better.

2 cups broccoli florets
1 cup pear, peeled and chopped
½ cup frozen peas

Place the broccoli in a steamer basket set over boiling water. Cover and steam 5 minutes. Add the pear and steam 2 more minutes. Add the peas and steam another 2 minutes.

Transfer to a food processor or blender and puree to desired consistency.

Yellow Lentils and Rice (Khichdi)

Makes 2 ¼ cups

Traditionally made with white rice, this dish is commonly used to wean babies in India, and is a good mix of protein and carbohydrates. You can use any type of rice, but brown rice is more nutritious. I like to use short grain brown rice because it cooks up softer, clingier, and mushier than long grain rice. Adjust the cooking time depending on what type of rice you use (white rice cooks faster). Yellow lentils are among the mildest and fastest cooking of all lentils. Rinsing them will help you to get rid of compounds that cause gas. Cumin aids in digestion, while turmeric has antioxidant and anti-inflammatory properties.

2½ cups water

¼ cup yellow lentils (moong dal), rinsed

¾ cup brown rice, preferably short grain

⅛ teaspoon turmeric (optional)

⅛ teaspoon ground cumin (optional)

I teaspoon butter (optional)

Bring the water to a boil in a medium saucepan. Stir in the lentils, rice, turmeric, and cumin. Reduce to a simmer and cover. Cook on low heat until lentils and rice are soft, about 40 minutes. Stir in the butter.

Puree to desired consistency using an immersion blender or food processor.

Apple Strawberry Compote

Makes about 1½ cups

This delicious compote tastes as good as it looks. Serve it alone or stir it into yogurt or oatmeal. You can even use it to top pancakes or waffles. This recipe works well with many other fruits besides strawberries, including other berries, apricots, peaches, or plums.

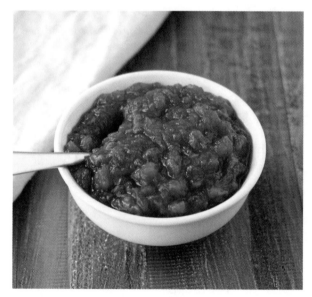

I large apple (8 ounces), washed, peeled, and chopped

1½ cups sliced strawberries

¼ cup water

Place the chopped apples, strawberries, and water in a medium saucepan. Bring to a boil then reduce to a simmer and cover. Simmer 15–20 minutes until fruit is tender.

Puree to desired consistency using an immersion blender or food processor or as your baby gets older, simply mash with a potato masher or fork.

Tropical Rice Pudding

Makes about 2 ½ cups

This dish is a nice twist on classic rice pudding—it uses coconut milk instead of cow's milk, and has no added sugar. Instead, it has natural sweetness from the coconut milk and mango puree. Coconut and mango are a natural pairing but you can use different fruit purees like cherry, apricot, blueberry, or banana.

½ cup basmati or jasmine rice
1 cup unsweetened coconut milk
¾ cup Mango Puree (page 105)

Place the rice in a medium saucepan with 1 cup water. Bring to a boil then reduce heat to a simmer and cover. Cook until rice is soft, 15–20 minutes.

Stir in the coconut milk and cook, on low heat, another 10 minutes until creamy. Stir occasionally to prevent scorching. Set aside to cool.

Puree with an immersion blender or food processor to desired consistency. Spoon some of the rice pudding into a bowl and stir in a dollop of mango puree. Store any remaining rice pudding and mango puree in separate containers and mix together when serving.

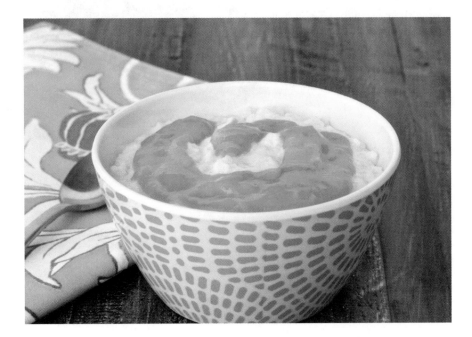

Purple Power (Blueberries, Kale, & Apple)

Makes 1¼ cups

This puree is a great way to incorporate nutritious greens like kale into your baby's diet. They'll love the flavor, as well as the vibrant purple color of this dish. Look for Tuscan kale (also called lacinato or dinosaur kale), which has a milder flavor and more delicate texture than curly kale. You can also use baby kale.

2 medium apples, washed, peeled, and chopped

1 cup chopped Tuscan (lacinato) kale, washed, peeled, and chopped

½ cup blueberries, washed

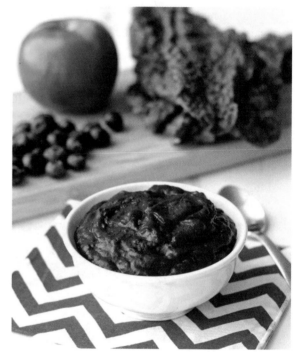

Place the apples and kale in a steamer basket set over boiling water. Cover and steam for 8 minutes. Add the blueberries and steam an additional 2 minutes (optional).

Puree with an immersion blender or food processor until smooth, adding a small amount of the cooking liquid if needed. If desired, strain the puree through a fine-mesh sieve. Cool and serve or store.

Orange Crush (Carrots, Mango, & Nectarine)

Makes 1¾ cups

Your baby will love this flavorful, brightly colored puree. Plus, it's packed with vitamin A, vitamin C, fiber, and antioxidants. It's also delicious stirred into oatmeal or yogurt.

2 medium carrots, peeled and diced
1 medium nectarine or peach, peeled and diced
1 mango, peeled and diced

Place the carrots in a steamer basket set over boiling water. Cover and steam 8 minutes. Add the nectarine and mango and steam an additional 4–5 minutes (optional).

Puree with an immersion blender or food processor until smooth, adding a small amount of the cooking liquid if needed. Cool and serve or store.

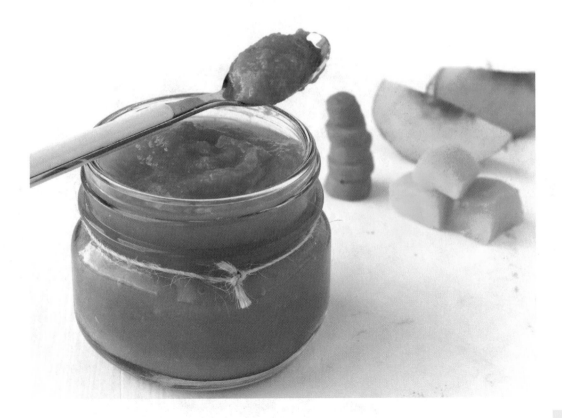

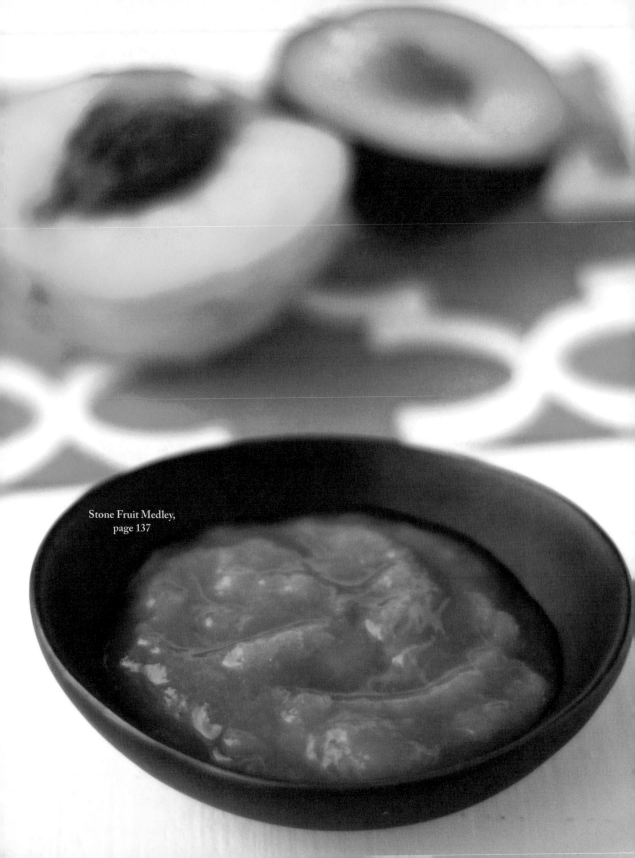

Stone Fruit Medley,
page 137

Roasted Recipes

ROASTING IS A COOKING technique that uses the hot, dry heat of the oven to cook food. It browns and caramelizes the surface of the food and concentrates the natural sugars in fruits and vegetables, intensifying their flavor. Roasting is an excellent cooking method for baby food because the food retains most of its nutrients, unlike some other cooking methods (like boiling).

Roasted Root Vegetable Trio

Makes 1½ cups

Roasting is an excellent way to cook starchy vegetables like sweet potatoes, parsnips, and carrots. If you're not familiar with parsnips, they look like white carrots but are starchier, similar to potatoes. They're easy to digest, and have a mild, sweet flavor that babies enjoy.

1 medium sweet potato, peeled	1 tablespoon olive oil
1 large parsnip, peeled	¼ teaspoon dried thyme or 1 teaspoon
1 large carrot, peeled	fresh thyme

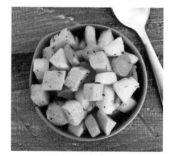

Preheat oven to 400°F.

Cut the vegetables into small pieces. Toss them with the olive oil and thyme and spread them out on a baking sheet in a single layer.

Roast in the oven until tender, about 20 minutes, stirring once halfway through. Puree or mash to the desired consistency for your baby. Or cut the vegetables into smaller pieces and let your baby enjoy them as finger food.

Roasted Bananas and Pears

Makes 2½ cups

Roasting isn't just for vegetables. Roasting fruit in the oven caramelizes their natural sugars and intensifies their flavors. It's also a great way to prepare baby food when you have fruit that's not quite ripe enough. Your baby will love this creamy puree, with its sweet, caramel-like flavor. You may have a hard time keeping your hands off it as well! Try stirring any extra puree into oatmeal or yogurt.

2 medium pears, peeled and cut into
wedges

2 medium bananas, peeled, cut into 2-inch
pieces and halved lengthwise

⅛ teaspoon cinnamon or cardamom
(optional)

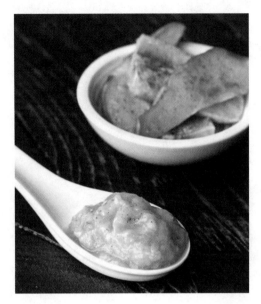

Preheat oven to 400°F. Line a baking sheet with parchment paper.

Place the pears and bananas on the prepared baking sheet and sprinkle them with cinnamon. Roast in the oven until they start to caramelize, about 20 minutes. Remove from oven and cool slightly.

Puree or mash to desired consistency. Cool and serve or store.

Stone Fruit Medley

Makes 1¼ cups

This dish takes advantage of the bounty of beautiful produce available at the markets in the summertime. Roasting stone fruit deepens their flavors and also makes it easy to peel off their skin. Feel free to use a mixture of peaches, nectarines, plums, and/or apricots. If you double the recipe, you can serve some of the roasted fruit to the rest of your family, topped with a dollop of yogurt.

2 peaches or nectarines
2 plums

Preheat oven to 400°F.

Cut the fruit in half and remove the pits. Place them in a baking dish cut side down and pour 1 inch of water into the dish. Cook in the oven until fruit is soft and skin is wrinkled, about 30 minutes.

Remove from oven and let cool, then peel off the skins. Transfer the fruit to a food processor or blender and puree to desired consistency.

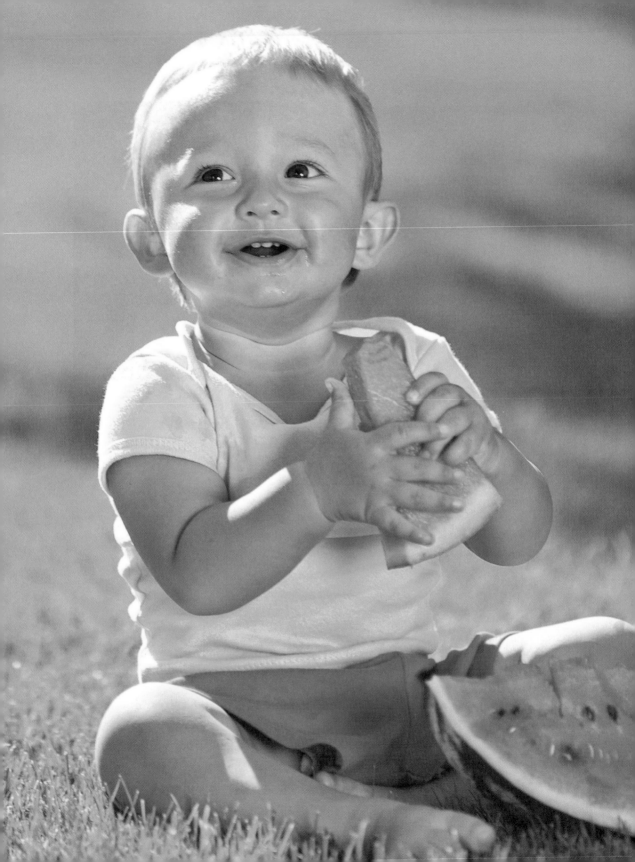

TASTY TEXTURES: 8–12 MONTHS

A FTER 8–12 MONTHS, YOUR baby has hopefully been introduced to a wide variety of foods and flavors. Now they're ready to move on to foods with thicker, chunkier textures. As she or he continues to grow, your baby is going to become a lot more interested in being an active participant at mealtime. Babies are now ready to start exploring the world of self-feeding, an important developmental skill. Have your baby join the rest of the family at meals as often as possible. At this age, babies enjoy being at the table; it's an important way for them to hone their motor skills as well as their social skills.

Your baby's mouth control and chewing ability is improving every day. Babies won't actually develop their molars until they're a little older, but they are very effective at mashing food between their gums. Start phasing out smooth purees and begin offering foods with a lumpier texture to encourage chewing. This textural variety helps babies learn to use their mouth and tongue, which in turn helps with speech development. Rather than pureeing food in a blender until completely smooth, start pulsing it in a food processor, or with an immersion blender (many foods can simply be mashed with a fork or potato masher). You can start introducing finely minced meat instead of pureed meat, as tolerated.

At this age, most babies will want to start eating independently, playing with their food and feeding themselves. Encourage this exploration of food and feeding utensils: give your little one a soft spoon to hold and practice with while you do most of the actual feeding. Just don't be surprised if half of the food ends up on the floor! Don't let the mess deter you; be patient, and invest in a drop cloth to put under the high chair (as well as a handheld vacuum cleaner!)

By 8–10 months, infants will develop the pincer grip, which allows them to pick up small objects between their thumb and index finger. Once this happens, it means that they're ready to try finger foods. Encouraging finger feeding helps your baby develop healthy, independent eating habits. Giving them a sense of control over what they eat will help them become more flexible eaters as they get older. It will also help them learn to regulate how much they eat.

Start introducing finger foods like soft, cooked pieces of carrot, O-shaped cereal, chunks of ripe pear, small pasta, or scrambled eggs. Babies also enjoy harder finger foods for teething like pieces of dry toast or bagel, rice cakes, or teething biscuits. Note that these harder foods should dissolve easily when gummed and melt in their mouths. Avoid foods that can be choking hazards, like whole grapes; whole nuts; raw, hard vegetables; large chunks of meat or cheese; and sticky foods like raisins, marshmallows, and candy. Refer to the Finger Foods section in this chapter (pages 171–177) for some recipe ideas.

Solids are going to become a large part of your baby's diet and at this age, you should have him or her on a regular feeding schedule that includes three solid meals a day. As your baby continues to grow, so too will their appetite. You can start offering two snacks a day: one in the midmorning and one in the midafternoon (some babies also needs a bedtime snack). Try to offer healthy snacks rather than reaching for packaged food.

Continue to offer a wide variety of nutritious foods, like fruits, veggies, protein, and whole grains. Continue to use herbs and spices to expand your baby's palate. You can use a wider variety of aromatics as well, like onions, garlic, and ginger, to add flavor to your baby's food. You should now be introducing combination meals to your baby, which combine grains, protein, and fruits or vegetables. Get creative with your combinations—your baby will enjoy the variety. Make dishes that have plenty of colorful, flavorful foods that they can pick up and eat, like Baby's Burrito Bowl (page 159) or Cheesy Quinoa Broccoli Bites (page 175). Many of the dishes in this chapter can be enjoyed by the rest of the family too: Baby's Bolognese (page 164), Chicken Corn Chowder (page 162), Risi e Bisi (page 158), and Creamy Split Pea Soup (page 155) are all good examples. Simply adjust the seasoning to taste once you've set aside your baby's portion.

Around this time, your baby can move on from a sippy cup to a cup with a straw to train a different set of muscles. Both of these types of cups are transitional; around 12 months, you can start teaching your baby to drink from an open cup. At this age, you can also introduce limited amounts of 100 percent fruit juice in a cup—but this should be limited to no more than 4 ounces per day. Juice does not have the fiber and other nutrients found in whole fruits and vegetables, and can be high in sugar. It's also less filling than breast milk or formula, so babies can overdrink it. Encourage water instead.

The following is a sample menu for an 8–12 month old. Remember that this is just a general guideline: the amount and types of food babies eat at each meal is highly variable. Also, don't worry about getting the perfect combination of foods in at every meal. Focus more on offering your baby a wide variety of healthy foods—the nutrition will balance out over time.

SAMPLE MENU FOR AN 8- TO 12-MONTH-OLD

MEAL	SAMPLE MENU	EXAMPLES USING RECIPES FROM THIS BOOK
Breakfast	· ¼–½ cup cereal or mashed egg · ¼ cup fruit · 4–6 oz. breast milk · or iron-fortified formula	· Peachy Banana Oatmeal (page 150) · Millet Porridge with Apples and Cinnamon (page 150) · Cherries, Butternut Squash and Millet (page 157) · Scrambled Egg with Plums (Pureed or Diced)
Mid-Morning Snack	· I serving grain · ¼ cup fruit or vegetable · 4–6 oz. breast milk or iron-fortified formula	· Teething Biscuit and Peaches or Pears (Pureed or Diced) · Classic Avocado Toast (page 210) · Pumpkin Banana Delight (page 126) on a Graham Cracker · O-Shaped Cereal or Pieces of Toast with Butternut Squash (Pureed or Diced)
Lunch	· ¼–½ cup protein* · ¼–½ cup vegetable or fruit · I serving grain · 4–6 ounces breast milk or iron-fortified formula	· Chicken, Mango, and Quinoa (page 160) · Baby's Bolognese (page 164) · Fish with Mushy Peas (page 166) and Basic Brown Rice (page 144) · Chickpeas, Spinach, and Pumpkin (page 155) with Barley (page 144) · Spinach and Ham Mini Frittatas (page 173) with toast
Mid-Afternoon Snack	· ¼–½ cup yogurt or cheese · ¼ cup fruit or vegetable · Water	· Yogurt with Mango (Pureed or Diced) · Strawberries, Beets, and Basil with yogurt (page 167) · Grilled Cheese Dippers with Creamy Tomato Sauce (page 173) · Cantaloupe, Peaches, and Cottage Cheese (page 128) · Sweet Potato Coins with Cheese (page 176) · Whipped Ricotta with Blueberries and Wheat Germ (page 168)
Dinner	· ¼–½ cup protein* · ¼–½ cup vegetable or fruit · I serving grain · 4–6 oz. breast milk or iron-fortified formula	· Chicken, Rice and Vegetable Dinner (page 161) · Salmon with Lentils and Carrots (page 166) plus Quinoa (page 146) · Beef and Barley with Pumpkin (page 163) · Stewed Pork with Apple and Sweet Potato (page 165) plus Basic Brown Rice (page 144) · Baby's Burrito Bowl (page 159) · Coconut Rice with Sweet Potatoes (page 158) plus Diced Tofu
Before Bed	· 6–8 oz. breast milk or iron-fortified formula	

Protein includes meat, poultry, fish, cooked legumes (like beans and lentils), tofu, and eggs

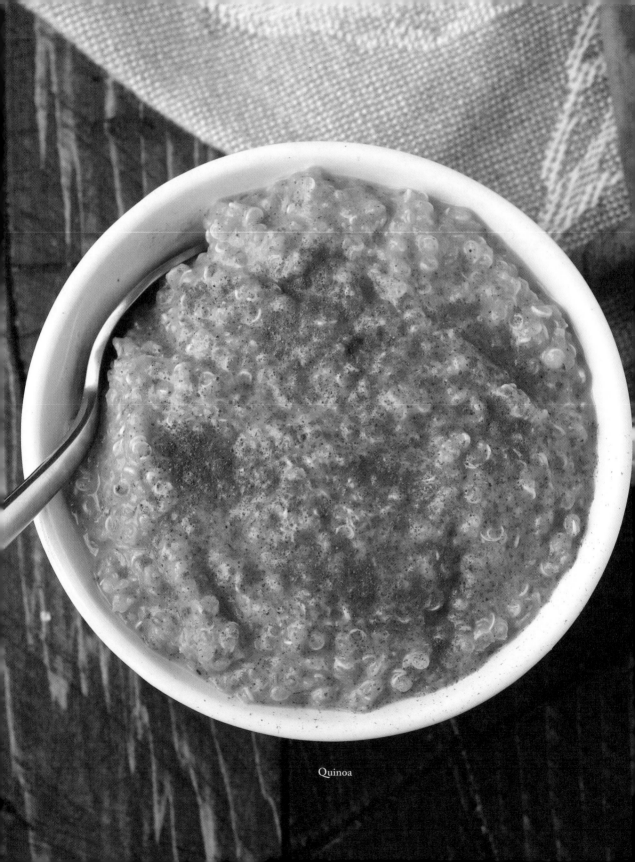

Quinoa

Great Grains

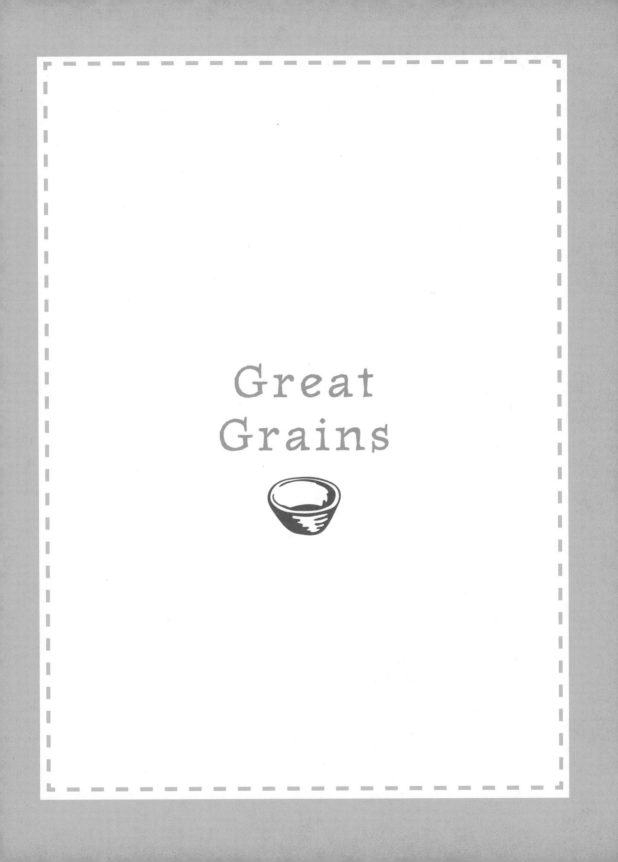

Basic Brown Rice

Makes 2 cups

Brown rice is a nutritious whole grain. It takes longer to cook than white rice, so make a large batch and freeze the unused portion. It's great to pair with many fruits, vegetables, and meat. It's also handy to have for quick, nutritious grown-up meals. I always keep cooked brown rice in my freezer. Look for short grain brown rice, which has a softer texture than long grain. Once the rice is cooked, you can puree it to the appropriate texture for your baby's chewing ability, or—eventually—leave it whole.

I cup brown rice, preferably short grain
2 cups water

Put the rice and water in a medium saucepan and bring to a boil.

Cover the pan and reduce to a simmer. Simmer until all of the water has been absorbed and the rice is tender, 45–50 minutes. Remove the saucepan from the heat and let stand, covered, for 5 minutes. Fluff with a fork before serving.

Depending on your baby's chewing ability, serve rice as is or puree in a food processor or blender with a little water to achieve desired consistency.

Barley

Makes 3 ½ cups

Barley is a nutritious whole grain with a slightly sweet, earthy flavor. Similar to brown rice, barley tastes good mixed with a wide variety of fruit, vegetables, and meats. Once the barley is cooked, you can puree it to the appropriate texture for your baby's chewing ability, or—eventually—leave it whole.

I cup pearl barley
3 cups water

Combine the barley and water in a medium saucepan.

Cover the pan and reduce to a simmer. Simmer until all of the water has been absorbed and the barley is tender, 40–50 minutes. Remove the saucepan from the heat and let stand, covered, for 5 minutes. Fluff with a fork before serving.

Depending on your baby's chewing ability, serve barley as is or puree in a food processor or blender with a little water to achieve desired consistency.

Oatmeal

Makes 2 cups

Oatmeal is a nutritious and tasty whole grain that's high in fiber and protein. It's classically mixed with fruit as a breakfast dish, but it can be served for any meal and pairs well with vegetables or meat. For an extra creamy treat, stir some yogurt into a mixture of oatmeal and fruit.

2 cups water
1 cup old-fashioned rolled oats

Place the water in a medium saucepan and bring to a boil.

Stir in the oats, reduce heat to medium-low and simmer until the oatmeal begins to thicken, about 5 minutes. Remove pan from the heat, cover, and let stand for 10 minutes until oatmeal is thick and creamy.

Thin the oatmeal with a small amount of water, breast milk or formula to achieve desired consistency. Depending on your baby's chewing ability, serve oatmeal as is or puree in a food processor or blender with a little liquid to achieve desired consistency.

Millet

Makes 3 cups

Millet is an ancient seed, and is a staple in many cultures, especially in Africa and Asia. Rich in iron, B vitamins, and calcium, millet has a mild corn flavor and is naturally gluten-free. Millet can be cooked to different consistencies—fluffy like rice, or creamy like oatmeal. Because the grains are so small, millet cooks up pretty quickly.

2 cups water
1 cup millet

Bring the water to a boil in a medium saucepan. Add the millet, cover the pan and reduce to a simmer. Simmer until all of the water has been absorbed and the millet is tender, about 20 minutes. Fluff with a fork before serving.

Quinoa

Makes 3 cups

Quinoa is a true superfood. It was so central to the ancient Incan culture that it was referred to as the Mother Grain. It comes in three main varieties: white, red, and black. Packed with vitamins, minerals and fiber, it is a complete protein, containing all nine essential amino acids, which makes it an excellent addition to a vegetarian baby's diet. Quinoa is also gluten-free and is tasty mixed with savory foods like vegetables, beans, and meat, or sweet fruits. For a creamier consistency, you can add a little breast milk or formula to the quinoa once it's cooked.

I cup quinoa
2 cups water

Rinse the quinoa thoroughly under running water. Put the quinoa and water in a medium saucepan and bring to a boil.

Cover the pan and reduce to a simmer. Simmer until all of the water has been absorbed and the quinoa is tender, about 15 minutes. Remove the saucepan from the heat and let stand, covered, for 5 minutes. Fluff with a fork before serving.

Depending on your baby's chewing ability, serve quinoa as is or puree in a food processor or blender with a little water to achieve desired consistency.

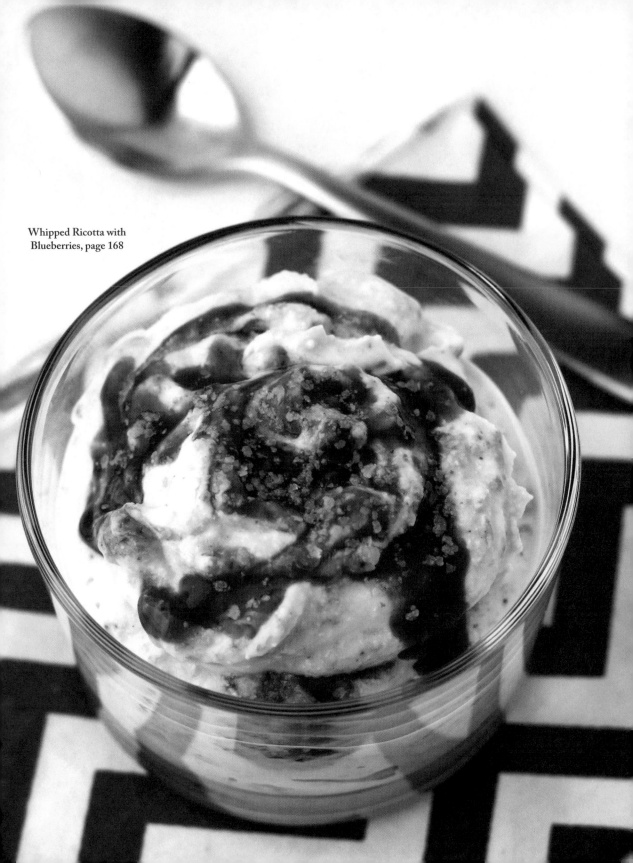

Whipped Ricotta with
Blueberries, page 168

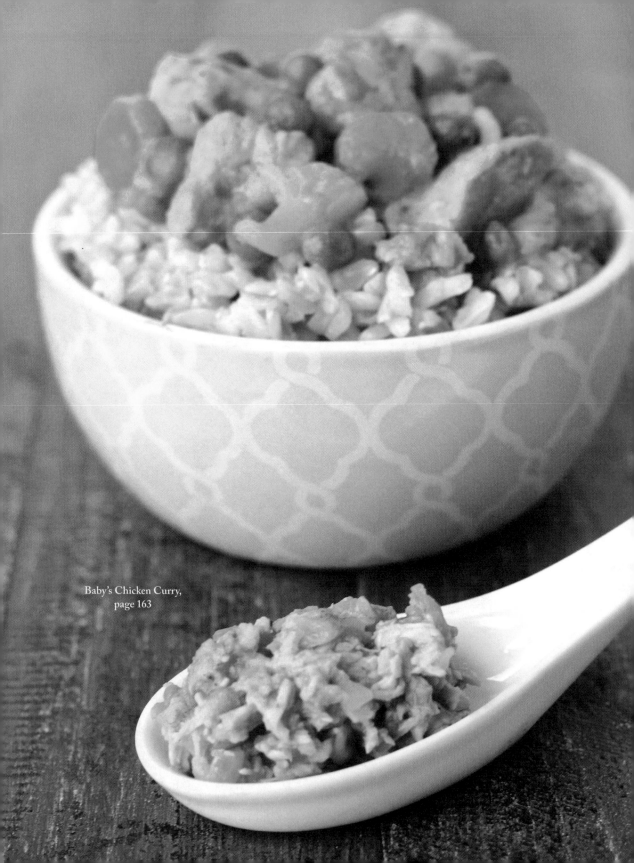

Baby's Chicken Curry,
page 163

Combination Meals

Peachy Banana Oatmeal

Makes ¾ cup

There are few things as comforting as a warm bowl of oatmeal for breakfast. Combined with fresh peaches and sweet banana, it's a hearty treat that your baby will love. Use this as a base recipe and substitute any combination of fruits that your little one enjoys. For extra creaminess, stir in some plain yogurt.

½ cup cooked oatmeal (page 145)
2 tablespoons peach puree (page 102)
½ banana, mashed

Combine all ingredients together in a small bowl. Depending on your baby's chewing ability, serve oatmeal as is, or puree in a food processor with a little liquid to achieve desired consistency.

Peachy Banana Oatmeal with Yogurt: Stir 2 tablespoons plain yogurt into the oatmeal and fruit mixture

Millet Porridge with Apples and Cinnamon

Makes about 2½ cups

Cooking millet in extra water gives it a creamy, porridge-like consistency. Your baby will enjoy the classic combination of sweet apple and warm cinnamon.

1 sweet apple like Fuji, McIntosh,
  or Golden Delicious
3 cups water

⅔ cup millet
¼ teaspoon ground cinnamon

Peel the apple and shred it using the large holes of a box grater.

Bring water to a boil in a medium saucepan. Add the millet, shredded apple, and cinnamon. Bring to a boil and then reduce heat to medium-low and cover. Simmer, stirring occasionally, until the millet is tender and creamy, about 20 minutes. If it seems to be getting too dry, add more water as needed to achieve a porridge-like consistency. Cool and serve.

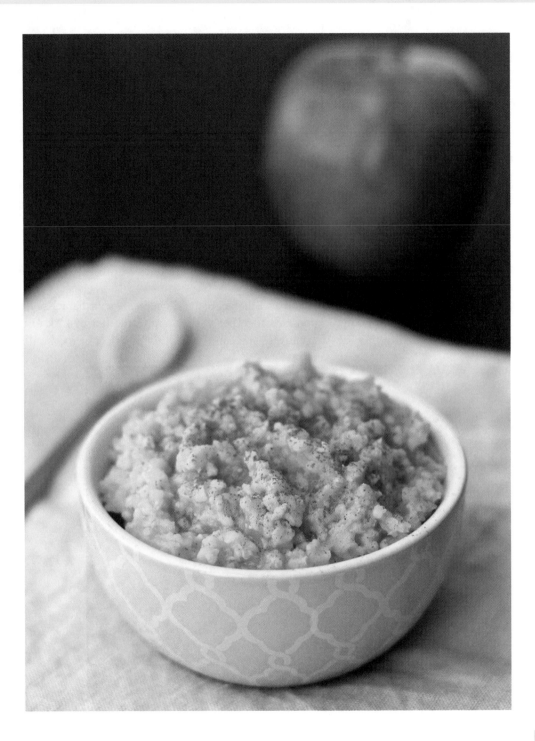

Jolly Green Baked Potato

Makes 2 cups

Combining broccoli with potato and cheese makes for a smooth, creamy, flavorful puree that your baby will love. Think of it as a baby version of a cheesy broccoli-stuffed baked potato. Potatoes are one of the few vegetables that don't puree well in a food processor or blender because the starch makes it gummy. You're best off mashing them, or else using a ricer or food mill.

1 large russet potato, peeled and cubed	2 tablespoons plain Greek yogurt
1 cup broccoli florets	¼ cup grated mild cheddar cheese

Pour water into a large saucepan to a depth of 1 inch and insert a steamer basket. Put the potatoes in the basket. Bring to a boil. Cover and steam for 5 minutes.

Add the broccoli and steam for an additional 8–10 minutes, or until vegetables are tender.

Transfer the vegetables to a bowl and add the yogurt and cheese. If your baby has the chewing ability, mash all of the ingredients together with a potato masher or fork until smooth or leave slightly chunky. Alternatively, you can run it through a ricer or food mill.

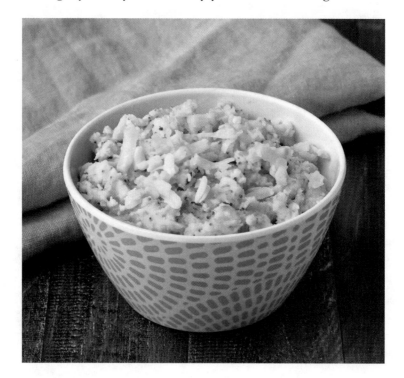

Baby's First Pasta

Makes I cup

Pasta can typically be introduced into your baby's diet around 8 months and up (unless there's an allergy to wheat). Pastina are tiny, dried pasta that come in a variety of shapes, including stelline, which are star-shaped. It's a common food for babies in Italy when first being introduced to solids. Pastina can be served plain, with just a little butter and grated cheese, or else it can be mixed with a fruit or vegetable puree or sauce. You can also stir in a little ricotta cheese for a creamier sauce.

- ⅓ cup pastina or other small soup pasta
- I teaspoon unsalted butter
- 2 teaspoons freshly grated Parmesan cheese

Cook the pastina according to package directions. Stir in the butter and cheese. Cool and serve or store.

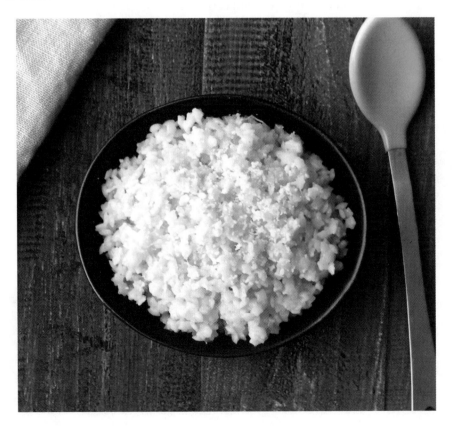

Pastina with Orange Sauce

Makes about 1 cup

This dish is loaded with important nutrients, including vitamin A, vitamin C, potassium, and fiber. Tomatoes are also a rich source of the antioxidant lycopene. Tomatoes used to be recommended only after age 1, but current recommendations give them the green light any time after 6 months. They are not highly allergenic, but may cause rash or mild digestive upset due to their acidity.

1 teaspoon olive oil
2 medium carrots, peeled and finely chopped or grated
1 cup tomato puree (no salt added)

¼ teaspoon dried parsley or basil
1 ounce (¼ cup) shredded cheddar cheese
⅓ cup pastina or other small soup pasta

Heat the oil in a small saucepan over medium heat. Add the carrots, cover and cook 5 minutes, until slightly softened. Add the tomato puree and parsley. Bring to a boil, then cover and reduce to a simmer. Simmer until carrots are soft, about 15 minutes.

Stir in the cheese until melted. Puree the sauce until smooth.

Cook the pastina according to package directions. Mix with the sauce. Cool and serve or store.

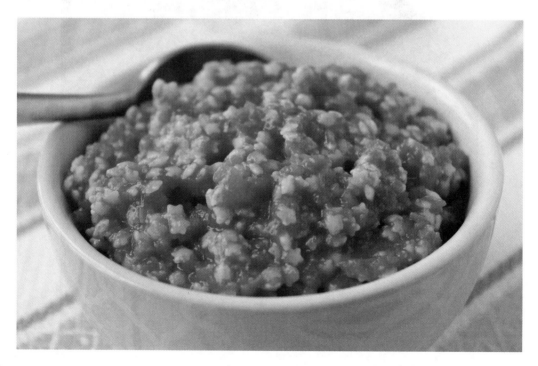

Chickpeas, Spinach, and Pumpkin

Makes 2 cups

This nutritious puree is packed with a wide variety of vitamins and minerals and chickpeas are an excellent vegetarian source of protein and fiber. This puree also works well with white beans in place of chickpeas.

> 2 cups baby spinach
> I can low-sodium chickpeas, rinsed and drained
> ½ cup fresh or canned pumpkin puree

Place the spinach in a steamer basket set over boiling water. Cover and steam until tender, about 5 minutes.

Transfer the spinach to a food processor along with the chickpeas and pumpkin. Puree to desired consistency, adding a small amount of water as needed.

Creamy Split Pea Soup

Makes about 4 cups

Split peas are inexpensive, easy to cook and packed with protein, fiber, and B vitamins. Babies will love the creamy, rich texture of this soup, which also provides plenty of vitamin A, vitamin C, and potassium. Double the recipe, and you have a light dinner for the rest of the family, too!

> 2 teaspoons olive oil
> 2 tablespoons diced leek or onion
> I medium carrot or parsnip, peeled and diced
> I small russet potato, peeled and diced
>
> I cup dried split peas, rinsed
> 3 cups water or low-sodium vegetable broth
> I bay leaf
> ¼ teaspoon dried thyme

Heat the oil in a medium saucepan over medium heat. Add the onion, carrot, and potato and cook a few minutes until they start to soften. Add the split peas, water, bay leaf, and thyme, and bring to a boil. Reduce to a simmer and cover. Cook until split peas and vegetables are tender, 40–45 minutes.

Remove bay leaf and puree with an immersion blender or in a standard blender to desired consistency. Leave slightly chunky for older babies.

Lentils, Leeks, and Squash

Makes 2¼ cups

Babies will enjoy this combination of protein-packed lentils and sweet butternut squash (you can also substitute sweet potato or carrots for the butternut squash). Leeks are a good way to introduce your baby to the onion family, as they have a very mild, sweet oniony flavor and a soft texture when cooked. If you're not familiar with them, they look like large, overgrown scallions. The white parts are tender but the green parts are very fibrous, so don't use them. Leeks tend to be very gritty, so make sure to clean them thoroughly.

2 teaspoons olive oil
2 tablespoons finely chopped leek, white
  portion only
½ cup red lentils, rinsed
1 cup peeled and chopped butternut
  squash

⅛ teaspoon ground cumin (optional)
2¼ cups low-sodium vegetable or chicken
  stock or water

Heat the oil in a medium saucepan over medium heat. Add the leek and cook 3–4 minutes until slightly softened. Add the lentils, butternut squash, cumin, and stock. Bring the mixture to a boil then reduce to a simmer and cover the pan. Simmer on low heat until lentils and squash are fully cooked, 20–25 minutes.

Puree or mash to desired consistency. Serve alone or with Basic Brown Rice (page 144).

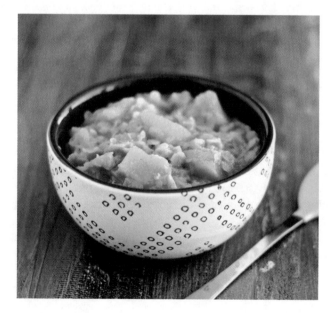

Cherries, Butternut Squash, and Millet

Makes 2 cups

Chunky purees like this are perfect for babies this age, as they learn how to chew. Bright orange butternut squash and ruby red cherries are chockfull of nutrients, including vitamin A, vitamin C, and antioxidants. Millet has a mild flavor that works well in this dish, but you can substitute other grains like quinoa, barley, or rice.

2 cups peeled and diced butternut squash
1 cup pitted cherries (fresh or frozen)
¾ cup cooked Millet (see page 145)

Place the squash in a steamer basket set over boiling water. Cover and steam for 15 minutes. Add the cherries and steam another 5 minutes, until tender. Remove squash and cherries from the steamer and cool slightly.

Transfer to a food processor or blender and puree until smooth, adding a small amount of water as needed to reach a smooth consistency. Stir in the millet. Serve or store.

For younger babies, puree to desired consistency.

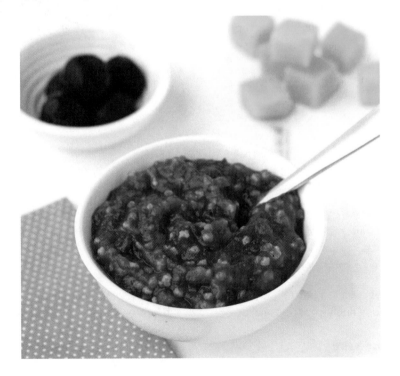

Coconut Rice with Sweet Potatoes

Makes 1¼ cups

Coconut milk adds a Caribbean flair to this yummy dish. It's a creamy combination of nutrient-packed sweet potatoes and whole grain brown rice that your baby will love. Be sure to set aside some for yourself too! For a boost of protein, add some diced chicken or tofu.

½ cup peeled, diced sweet potatoes
1 cup cooked brown rice
3–4 tablespoons coconut milk

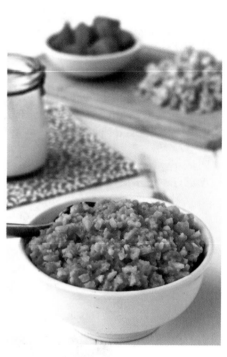

Place the sweet potatoes in a steamer basket set over boiling water. Cover and steam until tender, about 15 minutes.

Transfer the potatoes to a food processor along with the rice and pulse until coarsely ground. Add the coconut milk, one tablespoon at a time, and puree to desired consistency. Leave slightly chunky for older babies. Cool and serve or store.

Flavor boost: lime juice, curry powder, or ginger

Risi e Bisi

Makes 1½ cups

This is a traditional Italian dish of rice with peas. Arborio rice is a short grain rice and therefore cooks up softer than regular long grain rice. Shallots are a member of the onion family and are commonly used in French cuisine. They are good to use in baby food because they have a very mild oniony flavor with a hint of garlic, and they become meltingly tender when cooked.

2 teaspoons unsalted butter
2 tablespoons finely chopped shallot or
   onion
½ cup arborio rice

1½ cups low-sodium chicken or vegetable
   broth or water
½ cup frozen peas
2 tablespoons grated Parmesan cheese

Melt the butter in a medium saucepan over medium heat. Add the shallots and cook a few minutes until softened.

Stir in the rice and broth and bring to a simmer. Cover and cook 20 minutes, stirring occasionally, until rice is cooked. Stir in the peas and cook another few minutes until rice is soft and peas are heated through. Add more broth or water as needed to keep the rice a bit soupy. Stir in the Parmesan cheese.

Serve as is, or puree to desired consistency, depending on your baby's chewing ability.

Baby's Burrito Bowl

Makes 1½ cups

This is the perfect dish to for babies to practice their pincer grasp. Full of protein, complex carbs, and healthy fat, this dish packs a nutritional (not to mention a flavorful) punch! This tasty dish is meant for the baby, but the whole family can enjoy it.

½ cup cooked brown rice (page 144), warmed
¼ cup black beans, drained and rinsed
¼ cup cooked corn
1 teaspoon chopped cilantro

⅛ teaspoon cumin
½ medium Haas avocado, chopped into small pieces
2 teaspoons grated mild cheddar cheese

Mix the rice, beans, corn, cilantro, and cumin together in a bowl. Gently stir in the pieces of avocado. Top with cheese.

Let your baby enjoy picking up the food with their fingers and feeding themselves. If your baby is not ready for finger foods, transfer the mixture to a food processor or blender and puree with a little water or low-sodium chicken or vegetable stock to desired consistency.

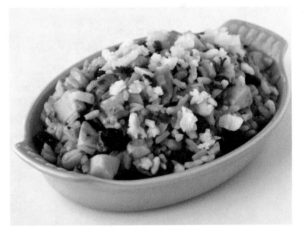

Cheesy Cauliflower Rice

Makes 2 cups

This dish combines nutritious whole grains and vegetables, while the cheese adds extra flavor, protein, and calcium. Use this recipe as a base and substitute any combination of grains and vegetables that you like.

  1 cup chopped cauliflower
  1 cup cooked brown rice (see page 144)
  ¼ cup grated cheddar cheese

Steam the cauliflower until tender. Reserve the cooking liquid.

   Mix the cauliflower, rice, and cheese together. Add a small amount of cooking liquid as needed. Puree or mash to desired consistency, depending on your baby's chewing ability.

Chicken, Mango, and Quinoa

Makes 2½ cups

This nutritious meal combines superfood quinoa with protein-packed chicken and sweet mango. Plus, the vitamin C in the mango will help your tot absorb the iron in the chicken.

  ½ pound cooked, ground chicken
  1 cup cooked quinoa (see page 146) or millet (see page 145)
  ½ cup Mango Puree (page 105)

Place the cooked chicken and quinoa in a food processor and puree to desired consistency, adding a small amount of water, breast milk, or formula as needed (depending on your baby's chewing ability, you may skip this step). Stir the mango puree into the chicken and quinoa mixture. Serve or store.

Chicken and Rice Dinner

Makes 2 cups

This combination meal provides a good mix of protein and whole grains. When your baby is ready, you can stir in a vegetable or fruit puree as well (suggestions are given below). As always, only introduce new foods one at a time and wait at least three days to watch for any reactions.

½ pound cooked, ground chicken

I cup cooked brown rice (see page 144)

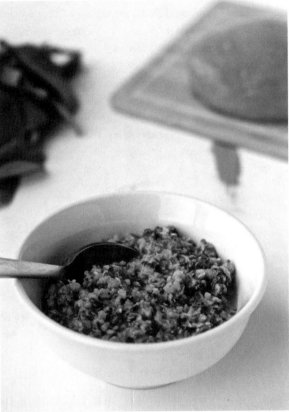

Place the cooked chicken and rice in a food processor and puree to desired consistency, adding a small amount of water, breast milk, or formula as needed. Stir in a vegetable or fruit puree, if desired (see below). Serve or store.

Chicken, Rice, and Vegetable Dinner variation: Stir ½ cup Sweet Potato Puree (page 68), Sweet Pea Puree (page 70), Carrot Puree (page 72), Zucchini Puree (page 72), Cauliflower Puree (page 97) or Spinach Puree (page 98) into the chicken and rice mixture.

Chicken, Rice and Fruit Dinner variation: Stir ½ cup Apple Puree (page 76), Pear Puree (page 77), Peach Puree (page 102), Plum Puree (page 103), Apricot Puree (page 104) or Mango Puree (page 105) into the chicken and rice mixture.

Chicken Corn Chowder

Makes about 3 cups

This tasty puree is packed with protein and complex carbohydrates. Dark meat cuts of chicken (like thighs and legs) have a higher amount of iron and zinc than white meat but either type can be used in this recipe. Sweet potatoes add a hint of sweetness and help give this puree a nice creamy consistency that your baby will enjoy. You may want to make a large batch of this dish, as it also makes an excellent soup for the rest of the family.

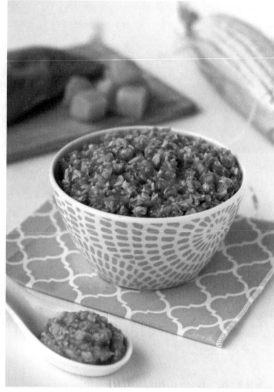

1½ teaspoons olive oil
2 tablespoons finely chopped leeks, white portion only (can substitute shallots or onion)
8 ounces boneless, skinless chicken thighs or breast, diced
1 cup diced sweet potato
1 cup fresh or frozen corn
1 teaspoon fresh thyme (or ¼ teaspoon dried)
1 cup low-sodium chicken broth

Heat the oil in a medium sauté pan over medium heat. Add leek and cook until softened, 2 minutes. Add the chicken and sauté 2–3 minutes. Add the sweet potato, corn, thyme, and broth.

Bring to a boil, and then reduce to a simmer and cover. Cook until potatoes are tender and chicken is cooked through, about 15 minutes. Cool slightly.

Transfer the chicken and vegetables to a food processor and puree, adding some of the cooking liquid as needed to thin the puree to desired consistency. Leave slightly chunky for older babies.

Baby's Chicken Curry

Makes about 4 cups

International dishes like this are a great way to introduce your baby to new flavor experiences. Curry powder is actually a blend of spices, and comes in a wide variety of spice levels—so be sure to choose a mild one for your little one. The curry powder in this recipe is nicely balanced by the naturally sweet, creamy coconut milk. Make extra and serve this dish to the whole family with brown rice or naan, an Indian flatbread.

2 teaspoons olive or coconut oil
2 tablespoons minced shallots, leeks, or onion
1 small clove garlic, minced
½–¾ teaspoon mild curry powder
2 teaspoons tomato paste
8 ounces boneless, skinless chicken breast, diced

1 carrot, peeled and thinly sliced
½ cup cauliflower, cut into small florets
½ cup unsweetened coconut milk
⅓ cup frozen peas
1 teaspoon chopped cilantro or basil (optional)

Heat the oil in a skillet over medium heat. Add the shallot and garlic and cook 1–2 minutes until softened. Add the curry powder and tomato paste and cook another minute until fragrant. Add the chicken and cook 2–3 minutes, stirring to brown it on all sides. Add the carrot, cauliflower, and coconut milk.

Bring the sauce to a boil then reduce to a simmer and cover. Cook 10–12 minutes until chicken is cooked and carrots are tender. Stir in the peas and cilantro and cook, uncovered, another 2–3 minutes, until peas are heated through.

Serve curry with Basic Brown Rice (page 144). Depending on your baby's chewing ability, either cut the chicken and vegetables into small pieces or puree to desired consistency in a food processor.

Beef and Barley with Pumpkin

Makes 2 ¼ cups

Pumpkins are very nutritious fruits (yes, they are fruits, not vegetables). They are loaded with beta-carotene, which gets converted to Vitamin A in the body. They're also a good source of potassium, protein, and iron. You can cook fresh pumpkin in the same way that you would cook butternut squash or acorn squash (see page 69). However, you can also buy canned pumpkin, which is a huge timesaver. Make sure you buy 100% pure pumpkin, not pumpkin pie filling, which contains sugar and other additives.

½ pound cooked ground beef
1 cup cooked barley (page 144)
½ cup canned pumpkin

Place the cooked beef and barley in a food processor and puree to desired consistency, adding a small amount of water, breast milk, or formula as needed. Stir the pumpkin into the beef and barley mixture. Serve or store.

Baby's Bolognese

Makes 2 cups

Introduce your baby to the flavors of Italy with this hearty and nutritious dish. While you're at it, make enough for the rest of the family to share. Bolognese sauce freezes well so make a large pot of it and freeze any leftovers. That way, you can heat it up anytime you need a quick and nutritious meal.

1 shallot or ¼ yellow onion, peeled
1 carrot, peeled
1 stalk celery
1 clove garlic
1 tablespoon olive oil
8 ounces lean ground beef
1 can (8 ounces) tomato sauce
    (no salt added)
½ teaspoon dried thyme
½ teaspoon dried basil
¼ cup low-sodium chicken stock
    or water
Cooked small pasta like ditalini,
    orzo, or mini shells
Grated Parmesan cheese for
    serving

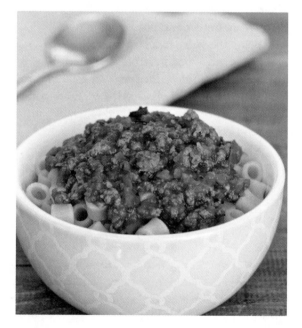

Roughly chop the shallot, carrot, celery, and garlic. Place them in a food processor and pulse until finely chopped.

Heat the oil in a large skillet over medium heat and add the chopped vegetables. Cook until softened, about 5 minutes. Add the ground beef and brown the meat, breaking it up with a spoon as it cooks. Add the tomato sauce, thyme, basil, and stock. Simmer the sauce 10–15 minutes until beef is cooked and sauce is thickened.

Let cool slightly, then pulse the sauce in a food processor or blender to desired consistency, if needed. Serve the sauce with pasta (depending on baby's chewing ability you may need to pulse the pasta in a food processor as well). Garnish with Parmesan cheese, if desired.

Stewed Pork with Apple and Sweet Potato

Makes about 3 cups

This dish takes the classic combination of pork chops and applesauce and adds nutritious sweet potato to the mix. Pork is a rich source of protein and also supplies several vitamins and minerals, including vitamin B12, iron, zinc, and selenium. Plus, the vitamin C in the apple and sweet potato will help your baby better absorb the iron in the pork.

8 ounces center-cut pork chop or pork tenderloin, diced
1 medium apple, peeled and diced
1 small sweet potato, peeled and diced

1½ cups low-sodium chicken broth or water
⅛ teaspoon dried sage (optional)

Place all of the ingredients in a medium saucepan. Bring to a boil, and then reduce heat to a simmer and cover. Simmer until pork is cooked through and sweet potatoes are tender. Cool slightly.

Transfer the solids to a food processor and puree, adding some of the cooking liquid as needed to thin the puree to desired consistency. Leave slightly chunky for older babies.

Fish with Mushy Peas

Makes about 1½ cups

Mushy peas are a common side dish in the UK, especially when served with fish and chips. Traditionally the peas are cooked down with butter until mushy and flavored with herbs like mint. In this quick version, the peas are mashed with butter and mint and then stirred together with fish and creamy yogurt to make a delicious meal for your baby. If you prefer, you can bake the fish in the oven rather than poaching it. To do this, place the fish in a greased baking dish, cover with foil, and bake at 350°F for 15–20 minutes until cooked through.

Water or low-sodium chicken or
  vegetable broth
6 ounces white fish filet like cod, tilapia,
  or flounder
½ cup frozen peas

1 teaspoon unsalted butter
1 teaspoon chopped mint or basil
3-4 tablespoons whole milk plain
  Greek yogurt

Fill a large saucepan or skillet with 1–2 inches of water or broth and bring to a simmer. Add the fish to the pan. Turn the heat to low so that the water is bubbling gently and cover the pan. Cook 7–10 minutes until the fish is opaque and cooked through. Drain the fish, reserving some of the cooking liquid. Flake the fish into pieces with a fork, checking for any small bones.

Meanwhile, defrost the peas according to package directions. Place the hot peas in a bowl with the butter and mint and mash with a potato masher or fork. Add the flaked fish and yogurt and mash to desired consistency.

Flavor boost: Add aromatics to the poaching liquid to infuse the fish with flavor. Try garlic cloves, chopped onion, sprigs of dill, or thyme or slices of lemon.

Salmon with Lentils and Carrots

Makes about 1½ cups

Salmon with lentils is a classic French pairing. Traditionally, French green lentils (lentilles du Puy) are used but you can substitute any type of lentils like red, yellow, or brown. Whatever type of lentil you choose, be sure to soak them first and then drain off the soaking liquid as this will get rid of many of the starches that cause gas.

1 medium carrot, peeled and chopped
1 (4 ounce) salmon fillet, skinned
½ cup cooked lentils (page 120)
⅛ teaspoon dried thyme

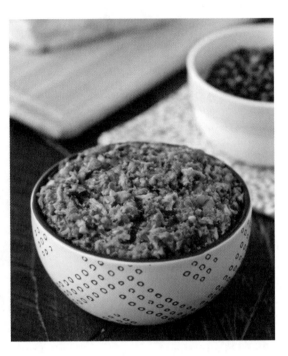

Place the carrots in a steamer basket set over boiling water. Cover and steam, 5 minutes. Add the salmon and cook another 6–8 minutes until carrots are tender and salmon is cooked through.

Transfer the carrots and salmon to a food processor and add the lentils and thyme. Puree to desired consistency, adding a small amount of water as needed.

Strawberries, Beets, and Basil

Makes about 1½ cups

This lovely magenta puree is rich in earthy flavor, antioxidants, and nutrients like vitamin C and fiber. Fresh basil adds a bright, herbaceous note, while Greek yogurt provides protein and calcium.

1 cup peeled, chopped beets
1 cup chopped strawberries
1 teaspoon chopped basil

2 tablespoons whole milk, plain Greek yogurt (optional)

Place the beets in a steamer basket set over boiling water. Cover and steam until tender, about 12–15 minutes. Remove beets from the steamer and cool slightly.

Transfer beets to a food processor along with the strawberries and basil. Puree until smooth, adding a small amount of fresh water as needed to achieve desired consistency.

To serve, stir together 2 tablespoons puree with 2 tablespoons yogurt, if using. Store the remaining puree.

Whipped Ricotta with Blueberries

Makes ¾ cup

Ricotta cheese has a mild, slightly sweet flavor that your baby will enjoy. It develops a fluffy, cloud-like texture when pureed in a blender or food processor. Mix it with blueberry puree for an out-of-this-world treat! Wheat germ adds fiber, protein, and a host of essential vitamins and minerals including vitamin E, folate, and zinc. This recipe works well with a wide variety of fruit purees, including cherry, peach, and mango.

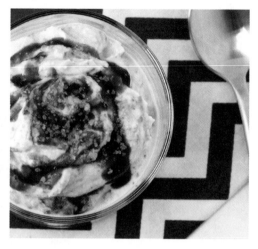

½ cup ricotta cheese
⅓ cup blueberry puree (see page 106)
1 teaspoon wheat germ (optional)

Blend the ricotta cheese in a blender or mini–food processor until fluffy. Or, whisk in a bowl until fluffy.

Mix the blueberry puree with the ricotta and stir in the wheat germ.

Hawaiian Sweet Potato Casserole

Makes about 2 cups

Nutritious sweet potatoes are combined with crushed pineapple and topped with a crumbly oat topping in this yummy dish that will make your house smell delicious as it bakes. If you use canned pineapple, be sure to get pineapple in 100 percent juice, not in syrup (which has added sugar).

1 large sweet potato, peeled and cut into small (½-inch) pieces
8 ounces crushed fresh or frozen pineapple (or 1 can crushed pineapple in 100 percent pineapple juice)
¼ cup old-fashioned oats, ground until finely chopped

1 tablespoon unsalted butter, cut into small pieces
⅛ teaspoon cinnamon
Optional: Greek yogurt for topping

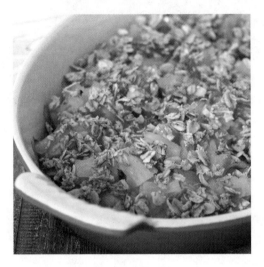

Preheat oven to 375°F.

Place the sweet potatoes in a casserole dish sprayed with cooking spray. Spoon the pineapple and juices on top of the potatoes.

Mix the oats, butter, and cinnamon together in a small bowl with your hands, until crumbly. Spread the mixture over the top of the potatoes and pineapple.

Bake in the oven for 25–35 minutes, until potatoes are soft. Mash with a fork or puree to desired consistency. Serve alone or with a dollop of yogurt.

Tropical Tofu Smoothie Bowl

Makes 2½ cups

Tofu is a great vegetarian source of protein. Its smooth consistency and mild flavor make it a good addition to many purees. Serve this dish right away or refrigerate it for later—the mixture will thicken in the fridge, giving it a nice custardy texture.

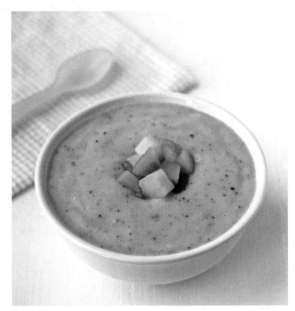

8 ounces silken tofu, drained
1 cup chopped, ripe mango
1 kiwi, peeled and chopped
½ banana

Blend all of the ingredients together in a food processor or blender until smooth. Serve or cover and refrigerate. Note that the mixture will thicken in the refrigerator.

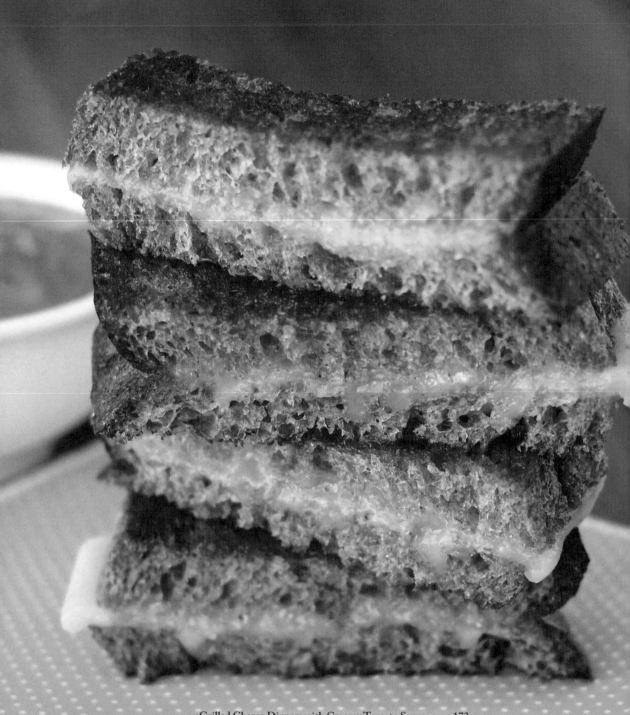

Grilled Cheese Dippers with Creamy Tomato Sauce, page 173

Finger
Foods

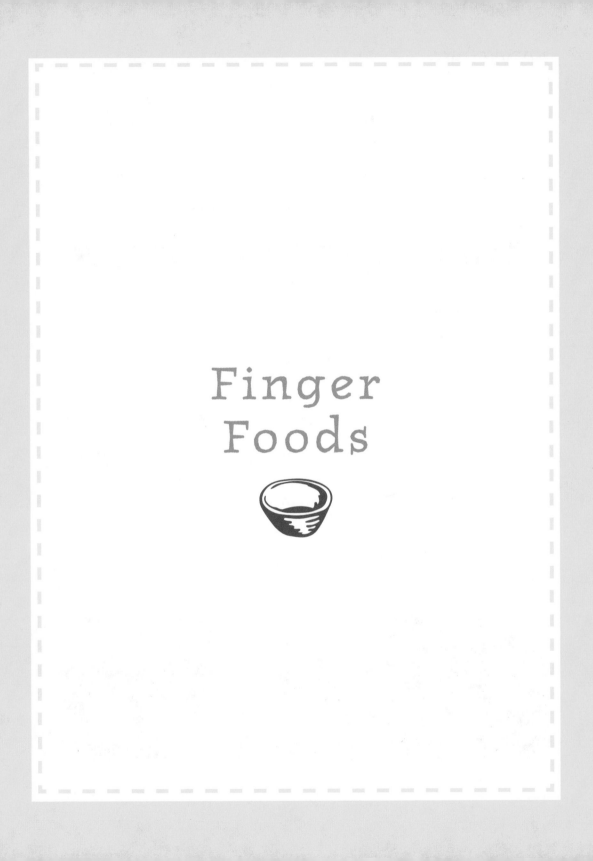

FINGER FOODS SHOULD BE cut into very small pieces, and should be soft or easily mashed between your baby's gums. You can coat finger foods with wheat germ or crushed cereal to make it easier to grip. As babies go through the teething process, they also enjoy some harder finger foods like pieces of bagel, rice cakes, or teething biscuits. These harder foods should dissolve easily when gummed, and melt in their mouths. Avoid foods that can be choking hazards like whole grapes; whole nuts; raw, hard vegetables; large chunks of meat or cheese; and sticky foods like raisins, marshmallows, and candy.

SIMPLE NO-RECIPE FINGER FOODS FOR BABIES

Fruits and Veggies	Grains and Legumes	Meat and Dairy
Soft, well-cooked pieces of sweet potato, carrot, or squash	O-shaped cereal (low-sugar)	Shredded cheese like mozzarella or cheddar
Ripe diced pears, peaches, or plums	Cut up pieces of toast or bagel (plain or spread with fruit puree, hummus, or nut butter)	Scrambled eggs (or yolks), diced hard-boiled eggs, or pieces of omelet
Steamed green beans	Small pieces of rice cake	Finely diced or shredded pieces of chicken or turkey
Ripe diced mango or papaya	Small, cut up pieces of pasta	Ricotta, cottage cheese, or cream cheese on cut up pieces of toast
Small, well-cooked broccoli or cauliflower florets	Diced pieces of tofu	Small pieces of cooked, low-mercury fish like cod, salmon, or tilapia (be sure to check for bones)
Diced banana or avocado	Small pieces of French toast, whole grain waffle, or pancake	
Chopped strawberries, halved raspberries, or blueberries (halved if large)	Well cooked lentils or halved beans (like black, white, or pinto beans)	

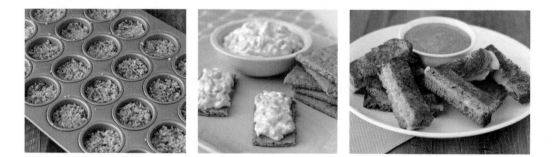

Grilled Cheese Dippers with Creamy Tomato Sauce

Makes 2 sandwiches

Filled with ooey-gooey melted cheese, your little one will love this classic childhood treat (and you'll have a hard time keeping your hands off, too)! Dip the grilled cheese sticks in creamy tomato sauce for the perfect finishing touch. Use whole grain bread for extra nutrients and make sure the cheese is cool enough before serving it to your baby.

Sauce
- 1 can (8-ounce), no salt added, tomato sauce
- 1 ounce cream cheese
- ⅛ teaspoon garlic powder
- ¼ teaspoon dried basil or oregano

Grilled Cheese Dippers
- 4 slices whole grain bread
- 1 tablespoon unsalted butter, softened
- 2 slices cheddar cheese

Place the tomato sauce, cream cheese, garlic powder, and basil in a small saucepan. Heat over medium-low heat until cream cheese is melted and sauce is creamy.

Meanwhile, heat a large skillet over medium heat. Spread some butter on one side of each of the four slices of bread. Place two slices of bread, buttered-side down, in the skillet. Arrange a slice of cheese on top of each one and place another slice of bread on top, buttered-side up. Cook a few minutes until golden brown, and then flip the sandwiches over. Cook another few minutes on the second side until bread is golden brown and cheese is melted.

Place the sandwiches on a cutting board and slice each one into 4 sticks. Let the sandwiches cool slightly before serving. Serve with creamy tomato sauce for dipping.

Spinach and Ham Mini Frittatas

Makes 24 frittatas

Perfect for small hands, these mini frittatas are a nutritious treat. Ricotta cheese makes the eggs nice and fluffy and adds a boost of calcium and protein. Spinach and ham are a perfect pairing, but feel free to substitute your favorite mix-ins like mushrooms, broccoli, bell peppers, sausage, or cheddar cheese.

4 large eggs
½ cup frozen, chopped spinach, defrosted and squeezed dry
½ cup ricotta cheese

¼ cup Parmesan cheese
¼ teaspoon garlic powder
½ cup (2 ounces) finely diced Canadian bacon or other lean ham

Preheat oven to 375°F.

Whisk the eggs, spinach, ricotta, Parmesan, and garlic powder together in a medium bowl.

Spray a 24-cup mini muffin tin with cooking spray. Sprinkle equal amounts of ham in the bottom of each muffin cup. Spoon the egg mixture into the muffin cups, filling them about three-quarters of the way full.

Bake in the oven for 12–15 minutes until they are puffed up and cooked through. Cool 10 minutes and serve. Extra frittatas can be stored in the refrigerator or freezer.

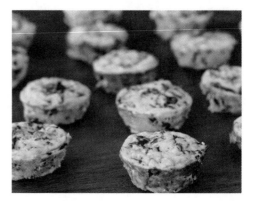

Pineapple Cream Cheese Spread

Makes about ⅔ cup

This simple spread is perfect for slathering on whole wheat toast, crackers, or graham crackers. Your baby will love the sweet flavor and creamy texture, and she or he will be getting a boost of vitamin C.

½ cup crushed pineapple*
½ cup (4 ounces) plain cream cheese
Whole wheat crackers or toast, for serving

Mix the pineapple and cream cheese together in a bowl until combined. Add some of the pineapple juice as desired to thin it out. Spread on crackers or toast.

*Mash fresh or defrosted frozen chopped pineapple in a bowl with a fork. If using canned, crushed pineapple, be sure to buy pineapple in 100% juice, not in syrup.

Cheesy Quinoa Broccoli Bites

Makes 24 bites

Packed with the superfoods quinoa and broccoli, these nutritious, bite-sized snacks will help satisfy your tot's hunger and give them long-lasting energy.

¾ cup quinoa
1½ cups water
2 large eggs
2 teaspoons Dijon mustard

5 ounces broccoli florets (about 1½ cups), steamed and finely chopped
1 cup shredded cheddar cheese

Preheat oven to 350° F.

Put the quinoa and water in a medium saucepan and bring to a boil. Reduce to a simmer and cover. Simmer until quinoa is cooked, 12–15 minutes. Set aside to cool.

Whisk the eggs and mustard together in a large bowl. Add the cooled quinoa, steamed broccoli, and cheese and stir to combine well.

Spray a 24-cup mini muffin pan with cooking spray. Spoon equal portions of the mixture (about 2 tablespoons each) into the cups and press down on them with the back of a spoon. Bake in the oven 17–18 minutes until cooked through and golden. Cool for 10 minutes, and then remove the bites from the pan and serve. Extra bites can be stored in the refrigerator or freezer.

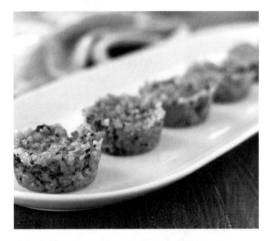

Sienna's Veggie Nuggets

Makes about 24 nuggets

Tasty, nutritious, and easy—these adorable nuggets were my daughter's favorite when she was younger. This recipe is a great way to incorporate a wide variety of vegetables into your baby's diet, and they'll enjoy picking the nuggets up and feeding themselves. Frozen vegetables are a great timesaver and make this recipe a cinch to prepare.

8 ounces frozen mixed vegetables like
   peas, corn, carrots, and broccoli
1 large egg
¼ teaspoon garlic powder

½ cup panko breadcrumbs, preferably
   whole wheat
¼ cup grated Parmesan cheese
1½ tablespoons olive oil

Preheat oven to 350°F.

Defrost the vegetables according to package directions. Puree them in a food processor until finely ground, but not totally smooth. Transfer to bowl and mix in the remaining ingredients.

Scoop heaping tablespoons of the mixture onto a greased baking sheet and flatten them slightly. Bake 20 minutes, and then flip and bake another 15 minutes. Cool and serve.

Sweet Potato Coins with Cheese

Makes about 40 coins

Sweet potatoes contain an impressive array of nutrients, including vitamin A, vitamin C, vitamin B6, manganese, potassium, and fiber. Slice them into thin coin-shaped pieces and roast them in the oven for a tasty and nutritious treat. Look for long, narrow potatoes, as they'll make smaller coins that will be easier for your baby to handle. A sprinkling of cheddar cheese adds flavor, as well as a boost of protein and calcium.

2 medium sweet potatoes (choose long,
   narrow potatoes), washed and peeled
1½ tablespoons olive oil

½ teaspoon paprika
4 ounces (1 cup) grated cheddar cheese

Preheat oven to 450°F.

Slice the potatoes into ¼-inch slices or "coins." Place them in a bowl and add the oil and paprika. Toss to combine well. Arrange the potato coins on a baking sheet lined with parchment paper. Roast in the oven for 10 minutes, then flip and cook another 10 minutes until tender. Remove the tray from the oven and sprinkle the coins with equal amounts of cheese. Return the tray to the oven and cook an additional 2–3 minutes, until cheese is melted.

Cool slightly before serving.

Zucchini Fries

Makes about 48 fries

Fries are the ultimate finger food! These healthy fries are made with zucchini, and are baked instead of fried. Before putting them in the oven, spray them with olive oil to get a nice golden color (an olive oil sprayer works best). You can try this recipe with other vegetables as well—eggplant, green beans, carrots, and celery root are all good options—you'll just need to adjust the cooking time.

¼ cup flour
2 eggs
1 cup panko breadcrumbs, preferably
   whole wheat
⅓ cup grated Parmesan cheese

1 teaspoon dried Italian seasoning
¼ teaspoon garlic powder
2 medium zucchini (about 1 pound), cut
   into sticks
Olive oil

Preheat oven to 425°F. Place a cooling rack on a baking sheet and spray or brush it with olive oil.

Prepare your breading station. Place the flour on a plate or shallow dish. Mix the eggs with 1 tablespoon water in a second dish. In a third dish, mix the breadcrumbs, Parmesan, Italian seasoning, and garlic powder together until well combined.

Working in batches, dip the zucchini sticks into the flour, shaking off any excess, then dip into the egg, and finally the breadcrumbs, coating all sides well with the mixture. Place the zucchini fries on the prepared baking sheet. Spray (or brush) them with olive oil.

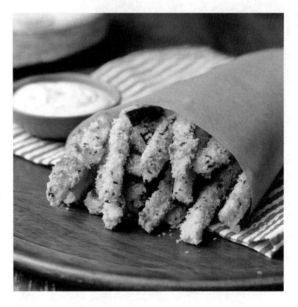

Bake in the oven until fries are golden brown and tender, 18–22 minutes. Cool and serve with your favorite dipping sauce or Greek yogurt.

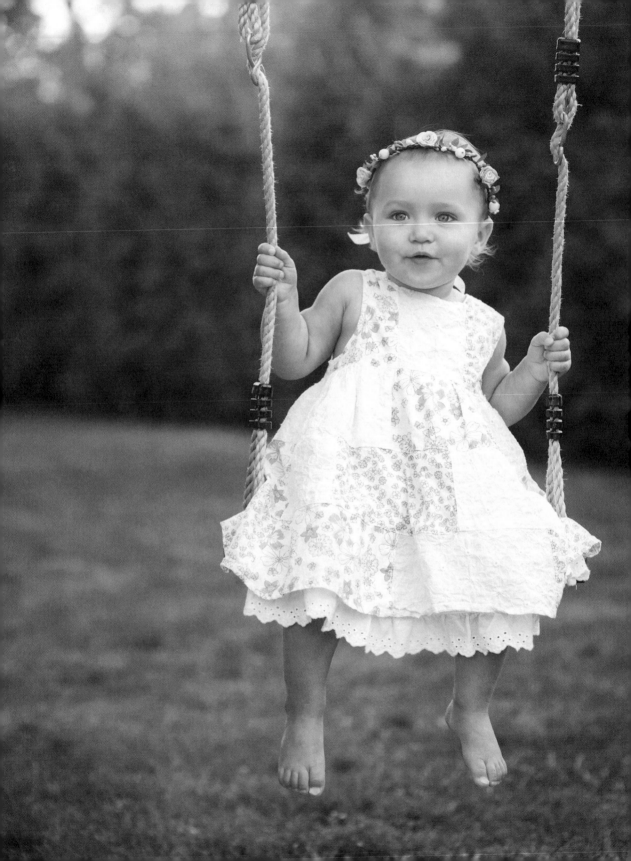

BIG KID MEALS: 12 MONTHS AND UP

THE TODDLER YEARS ARE a time of great transition, as babies begin to eat and drink more independently and continue to experience and accept new tastes and textures. It's also a transition for parents, as you start to leave bottles and purees behind and move on to giving your little one table food. If you haven't done so already, pull your baby's chair up to the dinner table so that they can join the rest of the family at meals. The recipes provided in this chapter are meant for the whole family to enjoy together. If your little one sees the rest of the family sharing a nutritious meal together, they will be more likely to want to eat it themselves. This is the best way to create good eating habits for life. It will also simplify mealtime for the cook! Just be sure to cut your baby's portion into pieces small enough for him or her to handle and adjust seasonings as needed (i.e. hold the cayenne pepper for baby's portion). Allow your little one to self-feed as much as they can—it's an important developmental skill.

Growth actually slows down once your little one becomes a toddler, but as they are more active now than ever, good nutrition is still a top priority! Toddlers' eating habits are notoriously unpredictable, but in general, after their first birthday, they'll need around 1,000 calories a day, depending on their age, size, and level of physical activity. This can be divided into three small meals and 2–3 snacks a day. However, don't get caught up counting the number of calories your tot is eating, and don't worry if they don't follow the same eating pattern every day. Some days they may eat a consistent amount at every meal, and other days they may choose to eat nothing for breakfast or lunch. They may love a food for a few days in a row and then completely reject it the next day. This erratic (and often frustrating) behavior is entirely normal, so remember not to take it personally. Try to avoid turning mealtimes into a battle—after all, the harder you push your child to eat a certain food, the less likely they are to comply.

Providing healthy snacks for your little one is a great way to help balance out an uneven diet. At times, babies may seem like they're too busy exploring the world to slow down and eat. This chapter provides plenty of nutritious snack recipes that will boost your toddler's nutrient intake and give them long-lasting energy throughout the day.

Parents of toddlers often worry that their child is not eating enough. The following table will give you an idea of how much of each food group your baby should be eating each day, but it's important to note that this is just a general guideline, based on the USDA MyPlate food guide for the average 2-year-old. For children between 12 and 24 months, diets are still in transition, and so these recommendations can be used as a guide, but are not set in stone. Remember not to worry if your little one doesn't eat the right amount at every meal: nutrition is about averages, so just try to provide a wide variety of nutritious foods and your child's diet will balance out over time.

DAILY FOOD PLAN

Food Group	Daily Amount	Notes	Serving Size Examples
Grains	3 ounces	At least half should be whole grains	The following are 1 ounce: 1 slice of bread; 1 mini bagel; ½ cup cooked rice; pasta, or oatmeal, or 5 whole wheat crackers
Vegetables	1 cup	Provide a wide range of colorful vegetables—dark green, red, and orange; beans and peas; starchy, and other	The following count as 1 cup: 1 cup cooked, mashed or diced vegetables (this includes legumes like beans and peas); 2 cups raw, leafy greens
Fruits	1 cup	Provide a wide range of colorful fruits; choose whole or cut-up fruit over fruit juice	The following count as 1 cup: 1 small apple, 1 large banana, or 1 cup sliced or diced fruit
Dairy	2 cups	Use whole milk dairy products after age 1 (unless directed otherwise by your doctor) and switch to low fat after age 2	The following count as 1 cup: 1 cup milk or yogurt, 1½ ounces hard cheese (like cheddar or Swiss), or ⅓ cup shredded cheese
Protein	2 ounces	Choose lean meat, poultry, beans, peas, nuts and seeds; eat low-mercury seafood twice a week	The following are 1 ounce: 1 ounce cooked meat, poultry or fish; 1 egg; ¼ cup cooked beans; or 1 tablespoon nut butter

Getting enough calcium and iron are still priorities. Once your baby turns one year old, you can introduce cow's milk. Milk will be an important part of their diet, as it provides calcium and vitamin D to help build strong bones. In general, whole milk should be given to children until they reach 2 years of age, as the fat is needed for normal growth and brain development. After age two, most children can be switched to reduced-fat milk. If there is a family history of heart disease or obesity, your doctor may recommend reduced-fat milk starting from an earlier age.

In addition to milk, now that your baby will be consuming less iron-fortified formula and cereal, it's important to include plenty of iron-rich foods in their diet, like meat, poultry, fish, enriched grains, beans, and tofu.

Around their first birthday, you should start to phase out the bottle. Your baby should be drinking from a cup, switching to an open cup as soon as they can handle it, usually before age 2. Water and milk are the best choices for drinks, and juice should be limited to 4 ounces a day.

One last note: your little one can still choke on large chunks of food, so make sure anything you give them is mashed or cut into small, easily chewable pieces. Although they may always want to be on the run, this kind of activity increases the risk of choking, so make sure they are always seated and supervised when eating.

SAMPLE MENU FOR A 1-YEAR-OLD	
MEAL	**EXAMPLES USING RECIPES FROM THIS BOOK**
Breakfast	· Sweet Potato Pancakes (page 188) with Sliced Bananas · Peaches and Cream Baked Oatmeal (page 192) · Cheesy Scrambled Eggs (page 190) plus toast and sliced strawberries · Pumpkin Spice Quinoa Porridge (page 194) plus ½ Banana · ¼–½ cup whole milk or yogurt
Mid-Morning Snack	· Yogurt with Fruit · Banana Date Oat Muffin (page 187) · Toast with Ricotta, Strawberries and Honey (page 211) · ½ English muffin or graham crackers with almond butter and sliced bananas · ½ cup whole milk or water
Lunch	· ½ Avocado Egg Salad sandwich (page 204) · Turkey and Hummus Pinwheels (page 206) · Pita Pizzas with zucchini and corn (page 208) · Crispy Tofu Nuggets (page 200) with Steamed Carrots Sticks · ½ cup whole milk
Mid-Afternoon Snack	· Diced or string cheese with diced vegetables or fruit · Zucchini Tots (page 198) · Very Berry Smoothie (page 216) · Avocado Yogurt Dip (page 213) with sliced bell peppers and cucumbers · 1 cup whole milk or water
Dinner	· Turkey Florentine Meatballs (page 228) with Veggie-Packed Tomato Sauce (page 229) and Pasta · Chicken, Broccoli and Rice Skillet Bake (page 230) · Barbecued Cheddar Mini Meatloaves (page 238) with Spinach and Artichoke Baked Potato Boats (page 248) · Turkey Sloppy Joes (page 235) with Cinnamon Roasted Sweet Potato Fries (page 255) · Salmon Cakes with Dilly Yogurt (page 244) and Bacon and Egg Quinoa Fried Rice (page 252) · Sweet Potato and Kale Quesadillas (page 247) with Green Beans and Sunshine (page 257) · ½ cup whole milk

This chapter is filled with a wide variety of recipes that are nutritious and packed with flavor. The recipes are divided into the following categories:

- ✿ Breakfast
- ✿ Lunch and Snacks
- ✿ Soups
- ✿ Dinner
- ✿ Sweet Treats

Because the dishes in this chapter are meant to be shared by the whole family, the number of servings provided for each recipe is given in terms of adult servings. Keep in mind, however, that the number of actual servings will vary depending on the amount of food your baby eats at each meal. Also, the nutritional information provided incorporates full-fat products like whole milk and whole milk cheeses. My hope is that you will use these recipes for years to come; once your little one passes the two-year mark, you can start transitioning to reduced-fat products.

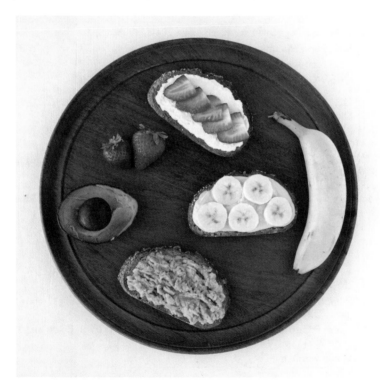

Strawberry and Cream Cheese
Stuffed French Toast, page 195

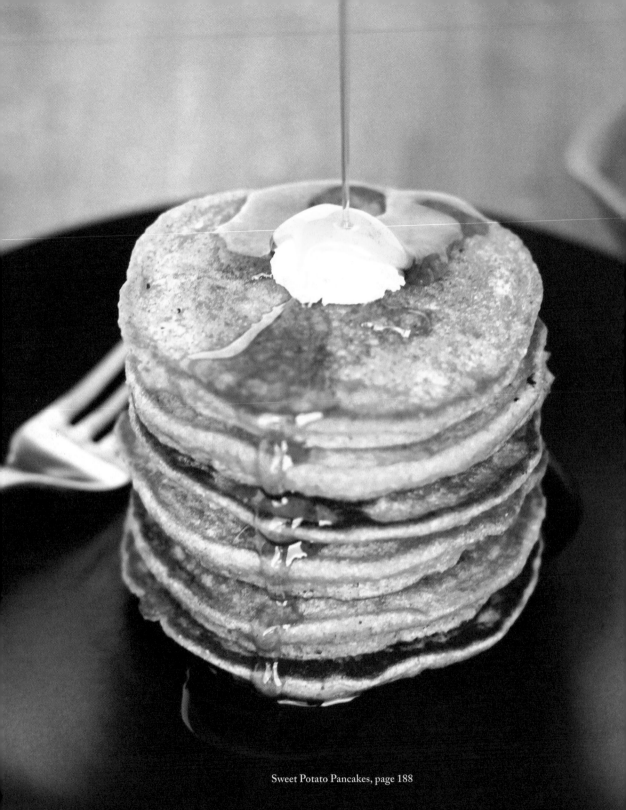

Sweet Potato Pancakes, page 188

Breakfast

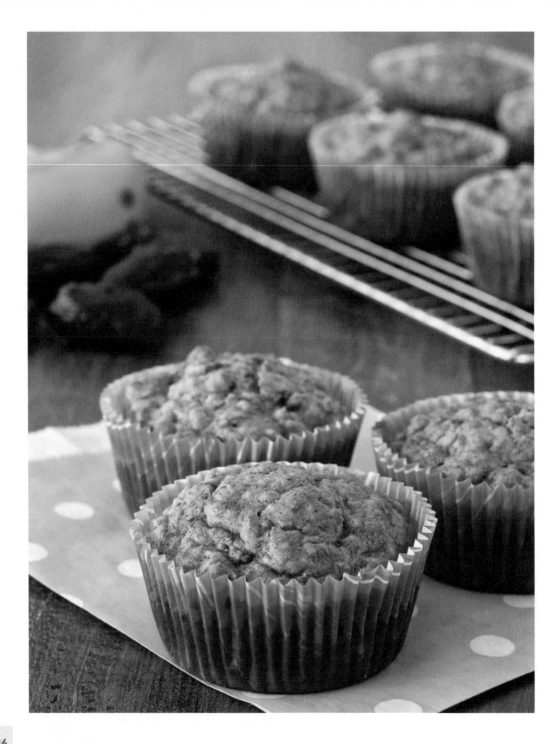

Banana Date Oat Muffins

Makes 12 muffins or 24 mini muffins

Made with nutritious whole grains and bananas, these delicious muffins are perfect for break-fast or a portable snack to take on the go. And the best part is they're naturally sweetened with dates—absolutely no sugar! Be sure to use really ripe bananas—the browner, the better—as they'll be sweeter. You can make extra date paste and use it to add a touch of sweetness to other dishes like oatmeal.

½ cup chopped dates (2½ ounces)
⅓ cup hot water
¾ cup all-purpose flour
½ cup white whole wheat flour
¾ cup quick-cooking oats*
2 teaspoons baking powder
1 teaspoon baking soda
½ teaspoon salt

1 teaspoon cinnamon
1¼ cups mashed, ripe banana (about 3 bananas)
1 large egg
½ cup milk
¼ cup neutral-flavored oil like safflower
¾ teaspoon vanilla extract

Preheat oven to 375°F.

Place the dates and hot water in a bowl and let them soak for 10 minutes. Puree in a mini-food processor until a smooth paste forms.

Whisk both types of flour, oats, baking powder, baking soda, salt, and cinnamon together in a large bowl.

Mix the date paste, bananas, egg, milk, oil, and vanilla together in another bowl (you can do this by hand or with a mixer). Add the dry ingredients to the bowl and stir everything together until just combined—do not overmix.

Spray a 12-cup muffin tin with cooking spray and spoon the batter into the wells. If using cupcake liners, spray them with cooking spray so the muffins don't stick. Bake in the oven 16–18 minutes until a toothpick inserted into the center of the cupcakes comes out clean. Cool muffins in the tin on a wire rack for 10 minutes before removing and serving.

NUTRITIONAL INFORMATION
One muffin: Calories 154; Fat 5.5g (Sat 0.8g); Protein 3.4g; Carbs 23.7g; Fiber 2.3g; Sodium 293mg

*If you don't have quick-cooking oats, you can make them. Simply pulse old-fashioned oats in a food processor until coarsely ground.

To ripen bananas quickly, place them in a paper bag and seal it the best you can. To ripen them even faster, place an apple or two in the bag. Apples and bananas both give off a lot of ethylene, which speed up the ripening process.

Sweet Potato Pancakes

Makes 16 pancakes

Your little one will flip over these pancakes! They're packed with whole grains and nutritious sweet potatoes, and flavored with cinnamon, nutmeg, vanilla, and a hint of maple syrup—perfect for Sunday brunch. If you can't find white whole wheat flour, use a mixture of whole wheat and all-purpose flours.

1 cup white whole wheat flour
2 teaspoons baking powder
½ teaspoon cinnamon
¼ teaspoon nutmeg
¼ teaspoon salt
1 large egg
¾ cup mashed sweet potato*

1¼ tablespoons milk
1½ tablespoons pure maple syrup
1 tablespoon melted coconut oil or
   unsalted butter
1 teaspoon vanilla extract
Oil or butter for frying

Whisk the flour, baking powder, cinnamon, nutmeg, and salt together in a bowl.

Whisk the egg, sweet potato, milk, maple syrup, coconut oil, and vanilla together in a second bowl. Add the dry ingredients to the wet ingredients and stir until just combined.

Heat a large skillet or griddle over medium heat and lightly coat with oil or butter. Pour the batter into the skillet, using about 3 tablespoons of batter for each pancake. Cook about 2 minutes, or until the pancakes start to bubble at the edges and the bottoms are golden brown. Flip and cook another 1–2 minutes on the second side. Remove from skillet and repeat with the remaining batter.

Serve pancakes plain or topped with butter and maple syrup.

NUTRITIONAL INFORMATION

One pancake: Calories 61; Fat 1.6g (Sat 1.1g); Protein 2.3g; Carbs 9.8g; Fiber 1.2g; Sodium 116mg

*A quick way to make mashed sweet potatoes is to cook them in the microwave. Place one medium sweet potato (8 ounces) on a microwave-safe plate and poke holes in it with a fork. Microwave 6–7 minutes until tender, flipping once halfway through. Cool and then cut in half and scoop out the flesh. Yields about ¾ cup.

Blueberry Dutch Baby

Makes 4 servings

Your family will rave about this lovely breakfast dish as it puffs up high in the oven. A Dutch baby, also called a German pancake, is a baked breakfast dish. Resembling a cross between a popover and a pancake, it has a light, tender, and eggy interior with crispy edges. Be sure to serve it right away, as it will start to fall soon after you take it out of the oven!

- 2 tablespoons unsalted butter or coconut oil
- 1¼ cup fresh or frozen blueberries
- 3 large eggs at room temperature
- ¾ cup milk
- ¾ cup flour (white whole wheat or all-purpose)
- ½ teaspoon vanilla extract
- ½ teaspoon cinnamon
- ¼ teaspoon salt
- 2 tablespoons coconut sugar or light brown sugar
- Optional: Blueberry Maple Compote (page 190), maple syrup, or lemon curd, for serving

Preheat oven to 400° F.

Place the butter in a 10-inch oven-safe skillet, preferably cast iron. Place the skillet in the oven for a few minutes until the butter is melted. Remove from oven and scatter the blueberries evenly in the skillet.

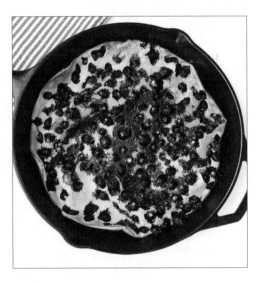

Blend the eggs, milk, flour, vanilla, cinnamon, salt, and sugar together in a blender until smooth. Alternatively, you can whisk the eggs and milk together in a bowl until blended and light yellow, and then whisk in the other ingredients until smooth.

Pour the batter evenly over the blueberries in the skillet and transfer the skillet to the oven. Bake 20–25 minutes until puffed up and golden brown. Remove from the oven and serve quickly (Dutch baby will start to fall within minutes of being taken out of the oven). Serve with a little maple syrup, Blueberry Maple Compote (page 190) or lemon curd, if desired.

NUTRITIONAL INFORMATION

One serving: Calories 268; Fat 10.2g (Sat 5.7g); Protein 9.1g; Carbs 33.1g; Fiber 3.9g; Sodium 220mg

Blueberry Maple Compote

Makes 1 cup

This quick and easy compote is the perfect topping for pancakes, waffles, or Blueberry Dutch Baby (page 189). Try it as an alternative to plain maple syrup. The blueberries add powerful disease-fighting antioxidants as well as vitamin C, vitamin K, and fiber. You can also use mixed berries, if desired.

1½ cups blueberries
2 tablespoons pure maple syrup
⅛ teaspoon cinnamon

Place all of the ingredients in a small saucepan and bring to a boil. Reduce heat to a simmer and cook for 5 minutes until the blueberries start to break down. Crush some of the berries lightly with a fork. Let the compote cool slightly before serving.

NUTRITIONAL INFORMATION
One serving (¼ cup): Calories 70; Fat 0.1g (Sat 0g); Protein 0.4g; Carbs 18.2g; Fiber 1.4g; Sodium 2mg

Cheesy Scrambled Eggs

Makes 1 serving

Don't skip the yolks when making eggs for your little one! Eggs are packed with beneficial nutrients for your baby and most of them (like vitamin D, choline, folate, and omega-3 fatty acids) are found in the yolk. Buy omega-3 enriched eggs for even more of this important brain-boosting nutrient.

1 large egg
2 teaspoons milk
½ teaspoon unsalted butter or olive oil

1 tablespoon shredded cheddar cheese
Pinch of kosher salt (optional)

Beat the egg, milk, and salt together in a bowl.

Heat the butter or oil in a small skillet over medium heat. Add the egg mixture and cook, stirring with a spatula, until large curds form. Add the cheese and stir until melted. Cool slightly and serve.

Southwest Breakfast Scramble variation: Stir any combination of the following ingredients into the eggs at the end when adding the cheese: black beans (drained and rinsed), chopped avocado, chopped tomato and/or chopped cilantro.

NUTRITIONAL INFORMATION

One serving: Calories 121; Fat 8.6g (Sat 4.5g); Protein 8.4g; Carbs 0.9g; Fiber 0g; Sodium 118mg

---

Breakfast Burrito Bites

Makes 8 bites

Your little one will love these playful breakfast bites. Eggs and bell peppers are wrapped up in whole wheat tortillas and cut into pieces like sushi. Simple, nutritious, and fun, this dish was shared by the talented Amy Roskelley and Natalie Monson over at the popular site Super Healthy Kids (www.superhealthykids.com). They note that eggs are an excellent source of important nutrients, including protein and choline, which is essential for your baby's developing brain. Bell peppers also add a boost of vitamin C, vitamin A, and fiber.

1 teaspoon olive oil or cooking spray
3 tablespoons chopped bell peppers
3 large eggs
1 tablespoon water
2 (8-inch) whole wheat tortillas

Heat ½ teaspoon oil in a nonstick skillet over medium heat. Add the peppers and cook until softened, 3–4 minutes. Remove peppers from the pan.

Whisk the eggs and water together in a bowl. Heat the remaining ½ teaspoon oil in the skillet and add the egg mixture. Cook the eggs without scrambling them. As they cook, move the edges inward until they're cooked all the way through, like a large fried egg. Flip and cook another minute or two on the other side.

Remove the egg from the skillet and cut it in half. Place one half on each tortilla. Add the peppers to the center of the tortillas and roll them up. Cut each tortilla into four pieces and serve.

NUTRITIONAL INFORMATION

One bite: Calories 65; Fat 2.7g (Sat 0.7g); Protein 3.4g; Carbs 6.9g; Fiber 0.8g; Sodium 109mg

Peaches and Cream Baked Oatmeal

Makes 8 servings

Oats and sweet peaches are baked together in this hearty and comforting breakfast dish that tastes so good it almost seems like dessert. You can substitute other fruits for the peaches—berries and bananas are excellent choices. Serve it alone or topped with milk, Greek yogurt, or a little bit of maple syrup.

2 ¼ cups old fashioned rolled oats

2 tablespoons plus 2 teaspoons coconut sugar or brown sugar, divided use

1 teaspoon baking powder

½ teaspoon cinnamon plus extra for garnish

¼ teaspoon salt

2 cups milk

1 large egg

2 tablespoons maple syrup

2 tablespoons melted coconut oil or unsalted butter

1 teaspoon vanilla extract

12 ounces (about 2 cups) diced peaches plus a few slices of peaches for garnish

Preheat oven to 350°F. Spray an 8 x 8-inch baking dish, with cooking spray. Mix the oats, 2 tablespoons sugar, baking powder, cinnamon, and salt together in a medium bowl. Whisk the milk, egg, maple syrup, coconut oil, and vanilla together in another bowl.

Scatter the diced peaches in the bottom of the prepared baking dish. Pour the oat mixture evenly on top. Pour the milk mixture on top and press to submerge all of the dry ingredients in the liquid. Arrange the peach slices on top and sprinkle with the remaining 2 teaspoons sugar and a pinch of cinnamon.

Bake for 35–40 minutes, until set. Let rest for 10 minutes before serving. Serve the oatmeal alone or top with milk, Greek yogurt, or maple syrup.

NUTRITIONAL INFORMATION

One serving: Calories 288; Fat 8.2g (Sat 4.8g); Protein 10.5g; Carbs 42.8g; Fiber 5.4g; Sodium 170mg

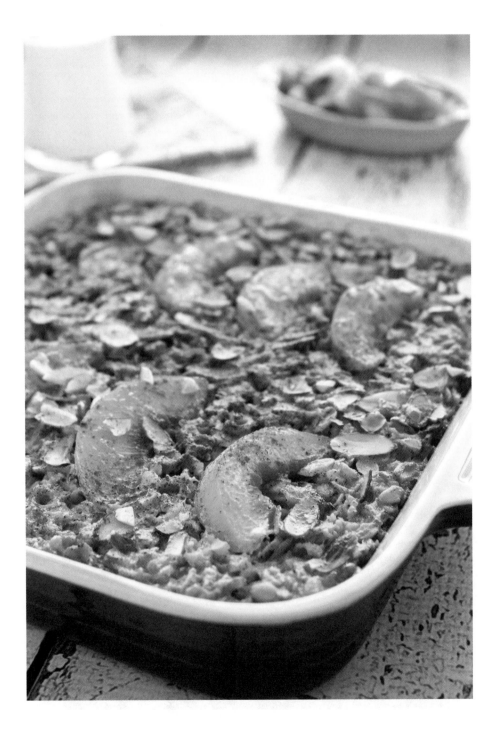

Pumpkin Spice Quinoa Porridge

Makes 4 servings

You and your baby can start the day off right with this nutritious whole grain breakfast. Quinoa is an ancient grain that's packed with protein, fiber, and plenty of vitamins and minerals. When cooked in a mixture of milk and pumpkin puree, it develops a rich flavor and creamy, porridge-like consistency.

I cup quinoa, rinsed
I cup milk
I cup water
½ cup fresh or canned pumpkin puree

I teaspoon cinnamon
¾ teaspoon ground ginger
I½ tablespoons pure maple syrup

Place the quinoa in a medium saucepan with the milk and water and bring the mixture to a boil. Stir in the pumpkin, cinnamon, and ginger. Lower the heat to a simmer, cover the pot and cook, stirring occasionally, until quinoa is cooked, about 15 minutes (it will have a porridge-like consistency).

Stir in the maple syrup, spoon the quinoa into bowls, and serve.

Note: The porridge will thicken once cooled so if reheating leftovers, stir in a little milk to loosen it.

NUTRITIONAL INFORMATION
One serving: Calories 225; Fat 4.2g (Sat 1.5g); Protein 8.3g; Carbs 38.5g; Fiber 4.3g; Sodium 32mg

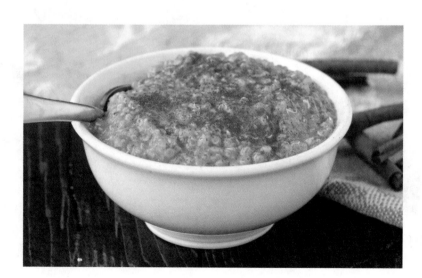

Strawberry and Cream Cheese Stuffed French Toast

Makes 4 sandwiches

This decadent treat is perfect for breakfast on a relaxing family weekend. French toast is stuffed with a creamy mixture of fresh strawberries and cream cheese. How can you beat that? Cut the French toast into triangles to make it easier for your little one to pick up and enjoy.

4 ounces (½ package) plain cream cheese, at room temperature
1 ½ teaspoons vanilla extract, divided use
1 teaspoon lemon juice
3 teaspoons light brown sugar, divided use
8 slices of whole grain bread

1 cup sliced strawberries, plus extra for garnish
2 large eggs
½ cup milk
¼ teaspoon cinnamon
Oil or butter, for the griddle

Mix the cream cheese, 1 teaspoon vanilla, lemon juice, and 2 teaspoons brown sugar together in a bowl. Spread equal amounts of the filling on each slice of bread. Arrange some strawberry slices on the surface of four slices of bread and top them with the other four slices of bread (cream cheese side down), forming four sandwiches.

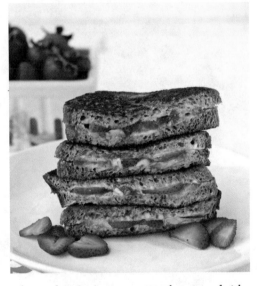

Whisk the eggs, milk, ½ teaspoon vanilla, and cinnamon together in a bowl or shallow dish.

Heat a griddle or large skillet over medium heat and brush with a small amount of oil or butter. Dip each sandwich into the egg mixture for a few seconds on each side and then place them on the griddle. Cook 3–4 minutes until golden brown, then flip and cook another 3–4 minutes on the second side.

Transfer sandwiches to a cutting board and let them cool slightly. Cut into triangles. Serve with fresh strawberries and a little maple syrup.

NUTRITIONAL INFORMATION
One sandwich: Calories 311; Fat 12.9g (Sat 7.1g); Protein 13g; Carbs 30.9g; Fiber 4.7g; Sodium 359mg

Zucchini Tots,
page 198

Lunch and Snacks

Zucchini Tots

Makes 16 tots

A fun take on a classic kid favorite, these tater tots use nutritious zucchini instead of potatoes. Zucchini has a high water content, so it's important to wring as much water out as possible to prevent the tots from getting soggy. These tots have Italian flavors and are delicious served with your favorite tomato sauce. Let your little ones have fun dunking them in the sauce.

1 heaping cup grated zucchini
¼ cup finely chopped shallot or yellow onion
¼ cup shredded mozzarella cheese
1 tablespoon grated Parmesan cheese
¼ cup whole wheat panko or other unseasoned dried breadcrumbs
1 large egg
1 teaspoon dried Italian seasoning
¼ teaspoon garlic powder
¼ teaspoon kosher salt
Olive oil
Veggie-Packed Tomato Sauce (page 229) or marinara sauce for serving

Preheat oven to 400°F.

Place the grated zucchini in cheesecloth or a kitchen towel and wring all of the excess water out (there will be a lot).

Place the zucchini in a bowl along with all of the other ingredients (except the olive oil). Mix until combined.

Line a baking sheet with parchment paper. Take a tablespoon of the mixture and form it into an oval shape. Repeat with the remaining mixture. Arrange the tots on a single layer on the baking sheet and spray or brush the tops lightly with olive oil.

Bake until puffed up and cooked through, about 20 minutes. Flip halfway through cooking. Serve with tomato sauce for dipping.

One tot: Calories 20; Fat 0.8g (Sat 0.4g); Protein 1.4g; Carbs 2g; Fiber 0.3g; Sodium 60mg

Asparagus in a Blanket

Makes 16 pieces

Vibrant green stalks of asparagus are wrapped in a blanket of puff pastry in this fun finger food. Asparagus is rich in several vitamins, minerals, antioxidants, and fiber. Cut off the woody, fibrous ends and peel away the tough outer layer to make it easier for your baby to enjoy.

1 pound asparagus (about 16 stalks)
1 teaspoon olive oil
Pinch of salt
1 sheet puff pastry, thawed

1 egg, beaten
Toppings: grated Parmesan cheese
(optional)

Preheat oven to 400°F.

Cut the tough ends off the asparagus. Using a vegetable peeler, peel the outer layer of the stalks. Toss the asparagus with olive oil and salt in a bowl.

Unfold the puff pastry on a lightly-floured surface. Cut the pastry into ½-inch strips. Wrap each strip around a stalk of asparagus, starting at one end and continuing down the stalk.

Arrange the asparagus seam-side down on a baking sheet lined with parchment paper or a nonstick silicone liner. Whisk the egg with a tablespoon of water in a small bowl. Brush the tops of the puff pastry with the egg wash. Sprinkle grated Parmesan cheese on top.

Bake in the oven for 15 minutes, until golden brown. Serve alone or with your favorite dipping sauce.

NUTRITIONAL INFORMATION

One piece: Calories 90; Fat 5.7g (Sat 1.5g); Protein 2g; Carbs 7.5g; Fiber 0.8g; Sodium 39mg

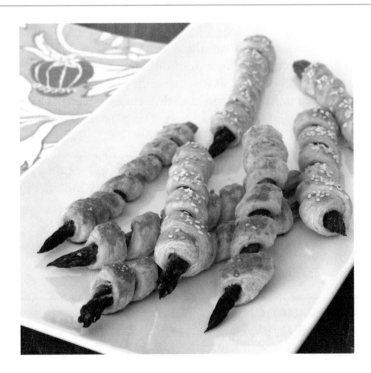

Crispy Tofu Nuggets

Makes 20 nuggets

This fun recipe is a healthier, vegetarian, baked version of the ubiquitous chicken nuggets that are on every restaurants' kids menu! Finger-licking good, these nuggets are made with nutritious tofu, which is packed with protein, calcium, and iron. This is an extremely versatile recipe and can also be used to make chicken or fish nuggets. Serve them with tomato sauce or your favorite dipping sauce.

I package (14 ounces) extra firm water-packed tofu, drained
¼ cup flour
I large egg
I cup panko breadcrumbs, preferably whole wheat
I teaspoon dried parsley
½ teaspoon garlic powder
½ teaspoon onion powder
½ teaspoon salt
2 tablespoons olive oil plus extra for brushing the pan
Veggie-Packed Tomato Sauce (page 229) or marinara sauce for serving

Preheat oven to 425°F. Brush a sheet pan with olive oil or spray with cooking spray.

Place the block of tofu on a plate lined with paper towels. Place another paper towel on top of the tofu and weight it down with one or two cans (canned tomatoes work well). Let stand for 10–20 minutes (this will drain all of the water out of the tofu).

Prepare your breading station. Place the flour in a shallow dish. Mix the egg with 2 tablespoons water in a second dish. In a third dish, mix the breadcrumbs, parsley, garlic powder, onion powder, salt, and olive oil together until well combined.

Cut the block of tofu in half crosswise, and then cut each block in half again. Cut each piece of tofu into five "nuggets." You should have 20 rectangular nuggets, each 2 inches by 1 inch.

Working in batches, dip each nugget into the flour, shaking off any excess. Then dip into the egg and finally the breadcrumbs, coating all sides well with the mixture. Place the nuggets on the prepared baking sheet. Bake in the oven for 10 minutes. Flip and bake for another 8–10 minutes until crispy and golden.

Let cool slightly then serve nuggets with tomato sauce for dipping.

Fish Nuggets Variation: Make fish nuggets instead, using the same method for pieces of tilapia, halibut, or other firm white fish.

NUTRITIONAL INFORMATION

One nugget: Calories 53; Fat 2.7g (Sat 0.4g); Protein 2.8g; Carbs 4.3g; Fiber 0.6g; Sodium 67mg

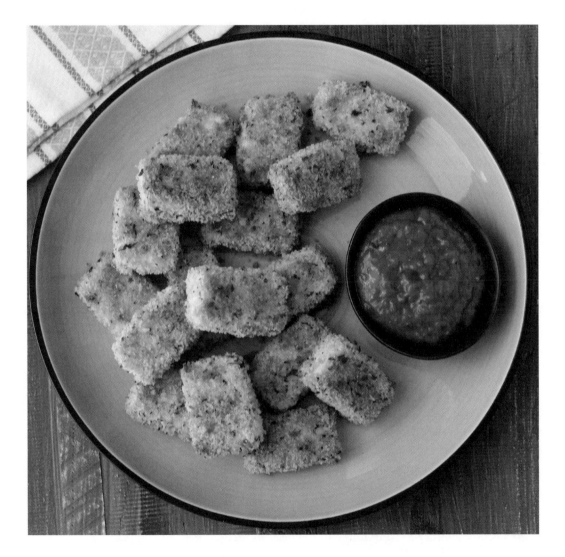

Cauliflower Cheesy Bread

Makes 16 breadsticks

Your baby won't be able to resist these healthy gluten-free bread sticks, made from cauliflower and topped with ooey-gooey melted cheese. Cauliflower is a cruciferous vegetable that's packed with powerful antioxidants, as well as an impressive array of nutrients. The cheese also adds a boost of protein and calcium.

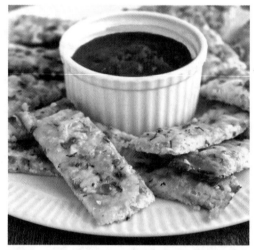

1 head cauliflower (about 2 pounds)
1 egg (or 2 egg whites)
1 cup shredded cheddar or Monterey
   Jack cheese, divided use
1 teaspoon dried Italian seasoning
¼ teaspoon salt
⅛ teaspoon pepper
Veggie-Packed Tomato Sauce (page 229) or marinara sauce for serving (optional)

Preheat oven to 450°F. Remove the outer leaves from the cauliflower and cut it into florets. Place the florets in the bowl of a food processor and pulse until finely chopped (it should look like rice).

Transfer the cauliflower to a microwave-safe dish or bowl. Cover and cook in the microwave for 10 minutes. Alternatively, you can steam the cauliflower in a steamer basket, or bake it in the oven at 375°F for 20 minutes.

When the cauliflower is cool, transfer it to a bowl lined with a kitchen towel or cheesecloth. Bring the ends of the cloth together and squeeze as much liquid out of the cauliflower as you can. Transfer the cauliflower to a mixing bowl and add the eggs, ½ cup cheese, Italian seasoning, salt, and pepper. Mix to combine.

Transfer the mixture to a baking sheet lined with parchment paper. Form the dough into a rectangle about 8 x 12 inches and ¼-inch thick. Bake in the oven for 15–20 minutes until cooked. Remove the baking sheet and sprinkle the remaining ½ cup cheese over the top. Bake for another 5–10 minutes, until cheese is melted.

Cut into 16 breadsticks. Serve with tomato sauce for dipping.

NUTRITIONAL INFORMATION

One breadstick: Calories 26; Fat 0.8g (Sat 0.4g); Protein 2.8g; Carbs 2g; Fiber 0.8g; Sodium 58mg

Goldfish Crackers

Makes about 400 crackers

Made with whole wheat flour, real cheese, butter, and a tiny bit of salt, these crackers taste better than their store-bought counterparts— and they're a whole lot healthier. Have fun making them with your children when they're old enough—they'll love playing with the dough and cutting out the adorable little crackers. Goldfish-shaped cookie cutters can be found online, or you can use any shape cutter you like. The number of crackers you get depends on how many times you re-roll the scraps.

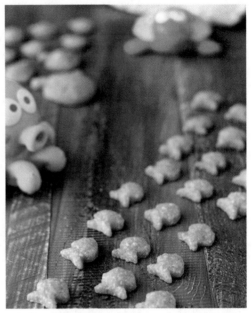

1 cup white whole wheat flour
½ teaspoon salt
4 tablespoons cold, unsalted butter, cut into pieces
8 ounces grated cheddar cheese
3 tablespoons cold water

Preheat oven to 350°F.

Place the flour, salt, butter, and cheese in the bowl of a food processor. Pulse until the mixture resembles a coarse meal.

Add the water, one tablespoon at a time, until the dough just forms into a ball. Remove the dough and place it on a flat surface, forming it into a ball. Flatten the dough into a disk, wrap in plastic wrap, and refrigerate for 10–20 minutes.

Roll the dough out to about ⅛-inch thickness. Cut out shapes using a goldfish-shaped cookie cutter (or any other shape cutter) and place them on a baking sheet lined with parchment paper.

Bake in the oven until crispy, about 15 minutes. Cool and serve. Store crackers in an airtight container.

NUTRITIONAL INFORMATION

One serving (about 1 dozen crackers): Calories 49; Fat 3.3g (Sat 2.2g); Protein 2.1g; Carbs 2.6g; Fiber 0.4g; Sodium 73mg

White Whole Wheat Flour

White whole wheat flour is a whole grain product that has all of the nutritional benefits of traditional whole wheat, but with a lighter color and milder taste (similar to all-purpose flour). It's milled from mild white wheat instead of red wheat, which can have a slightly bitter taste. White whole wheat flour also bakes lighter in texture than traditional whole wheat flour so it's a great choice for baked goods like these crackers.

Avocado Egg Salad

Makes about 1½ cups or 4 servings

Avocado and Greek yogurt replace mayonnaise in this nutritious and delicious egg salad recipe. It's packed with protein, healthy fats and a wide variety of essential vitamins and minerals. Your baby will love eating this rich, creamy dish by itself or spread onto whole grain bread or crackers.

4 large eggs
1 small, ripe avocado, peeled and pitted
1 tablespoon plain Greek yogurt
1 teaspoon fresh lemon juice
½ teaspoon Dijon mustard

1 tablespoon chopped, fresh parsley
Salt and pepper, to taste
Whole grain bread or crackers, for
  serving (optional)

Place the eggs in a medium saucepan and fill the pan with enough water to cover them by an inch. Bring the water to a boil. Once the water is boiling, remove the pan from the heat and cover the pan. After 12 minutes, drain the eggs and place them in a bowl of ice water for a few minutes. Then, remove the eggs from the water and peel them. Slice the eggs in half lengthwise and remove the yolks, placing them in a bowl.

Using a fork, mash the yolks with the avocado, yogurt, lemon juice, mustard, parsley, and a pinch of salt and pepper until smooth and creamy.

Finely chop the egg whites and add them to the bowl. Stir to combine. Adjust seasoning to taste. Serve on whole grain bread or crackers.

NUTRITIONAL INFORMATION

One serving (salad only): Calories 132; Fat 9.2g; (Sat 2.4g); Protein 7.1g; Carbs 3.7g; Fiber 2.4g; Sodium 163mg

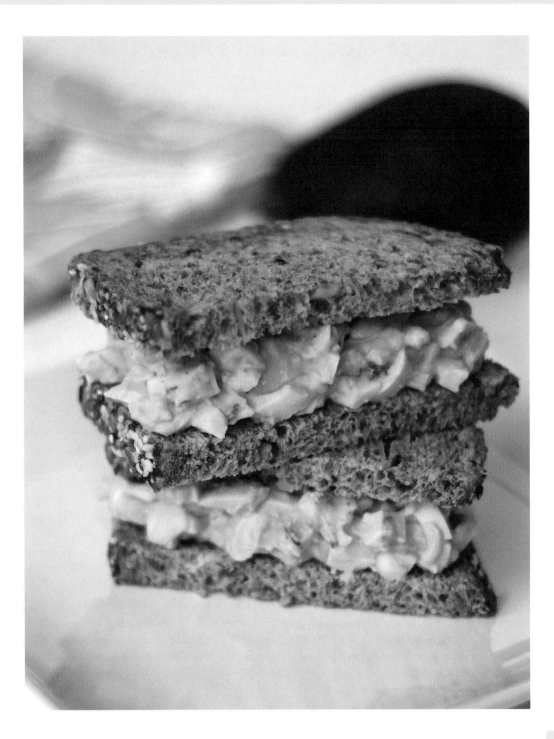

Turkey and Hummus Pinwheels

Makes 5 pinwheels

Children love foods that come in interesting shapes. Try making these pinwheels instead of the usual turkey sandwich. Simply spread hummus on a tortilla and pile on sliced turkey and a variety of colorful vegetables. Roll it all up like a burrito, cut into slices, and serve. You can make all sorts of pinwheels, using whatever ingredients you have on hand. I also make a Tex-Mex version with cream cheese, salsa, shredded chicken, cheese, and scallions. Or, you could try a sweet version with peanut butter, sliced bananas, and honey.

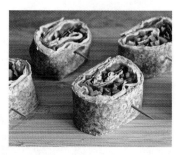

I large whole wheat tortilla
3 tablespoons hummus (see Classic
   Hummus page 214)

I ounce sliced deli turkey breast
¼ cup baby spinach leaves
¼ cup thinly sliced red bell pepper strips

Lay the tortilla out on a cutting board. Spread the hummus over the surface of the tortilla, leaving a one-inch border. Arrange the turkey slices on top of the hummus and sprinkle the spinach and pepper strips on top.

Fold in the sides of the tortilla and roll it up like a burrito. Use toothpicks to secure the filling in place and slice into five pieces. Remove toothpicks before serving.

NUTRITIONAL INFORMATION

One pinwheel: Calories 48; Fat 1.2g; (Sat 0.1g); Protein 3.1g; Carbs 6.7g; Fiber 2.4g; Sodium 144mg

Easy Soba Noodles

Makes 4 servings

This yummy noodle dish was shared by my fellow food blogger Alice Choi over at Hip Foodie Mom (www.hipfoodiemom.com). It's a super quick and easy dish that's perfect for a healthy mid-afternoon snack. When your children get a little older, it makes a great addition to their lunchboxes. Soba noodles are made from buckwheat flour and are gluten-free (check the labels, as some brands also contain wheat flour). They have a mild, nutty flavor and cook in just a few minutes.

4 ounces soba noodles

1½ tablespoons low-sodium soy sauce

1 tablespoon sesame oil

2 teaspoons brown sugar

Sliced cucumbers (can substitute other vegetables like bell peppers, snow peas, or broccoli)

Cook soba noodles according to package directions. Rinse with water, drain well and set aside.

Whisk the soy sauce, sesame oil, and brown sugar together in a small bowl. Pour the mixture over the soba noodles and mix well. Top with the cucumbers (or other vegetables) and serve.

NUTRITIONAL INFORMATION

One serving: Calories 135; Fat 3.4g; (Sat 0.5g); Protein 4.5g; Carbs 23.6g; Fiber 0.1g; Sodium 424mg

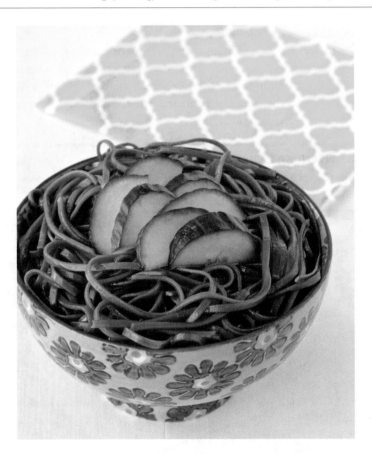

Pita Pizzas

Makes I pizza

Kids love pizza, and this is a quick and easy version that can be made in the toaster oven. Perfect for snacks, pizzas are also a great canvas for introducing nutritious ingredients to your young children. As they get older, they can help you in the kitchen and choose their own toppings. Slice the vegetables thinly or else chop them into small pieces so that they'll cook quickly.

I small whole grain pita
2 tablespoons low-sodium jarred tomato sauce
2 tablespoons shredded mozzarella cheese

Assorted sliced or chopped vegetables (like bell peppers, mushrooms, zucchini, spinach, or corn) or cooked chicken breast or shrimp
Olive oil spray

Preheat the oven or toaster oven to 400°F.

Place the pita on a baking sheet lined with parchment paper or foil. Spread the tomato sauce over the surface of the pita, leaving a border around the edges. Sprinkle the cheese over the sauce. Add assorted toppings of your choice to each pita. Spray the pizzas lightly with olive oil spray. Bake in the oven until cheese is melted and vegetables are cooked, 8–10 minutes. Remove from oven, cut and serve.

NUTRITIONAL INFORMATION

One pizza: Calories 123; Fat 3.4g; (Sat 2g); Protein 6.3g; Carbs 17.3g; Fiber 2.5g; Sodium 395mg

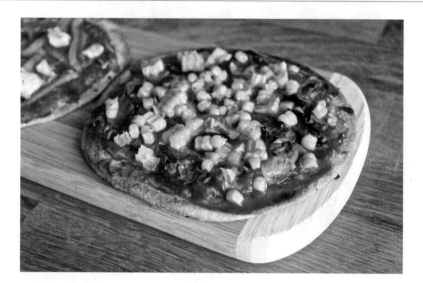

Pumpkin Banana Snack Bites

Makes 16–18 bites

This recipe comes courtesy of my friend Katie Serbinski, a registered dietician, mom, and founder of the blog Mom to Mom Nutrition (www.momtomomnutrition. com). She created these wholesome, nutritious, gluten-free bites as a healthy snack for her son. Baked in a mini muffin tin, they're perfectly proportioned for little mouths. Plus, they won't ruin anyone's appetite for dinner! If your child has a peanut allergy, you can substitute any nut butter, such as almond butter.

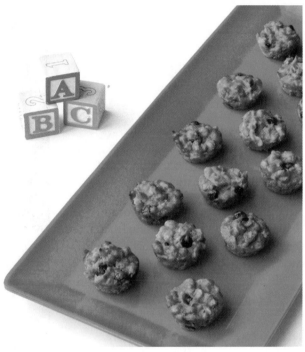

½ cup canned pumpkin puree
½ cup peanut butter
I medium ripe banana, mashed
½ cup old-fashioned oats
I egg
I tablespoon honey
I teaspoon vanilla extract
¼ cup chocolate chips (can substitute chopped dried fruit like cranberries or dates)

Preheat oven to 375°F.

In a large mixing bowl, combine all of the ingredients and mix well. Spoon the batter into a greased mini muffin tin.

Bake in the oven for 20 minutes until cooked through. Cool and serve (the bites can also be frozen).

NUTRITIONAL INFORMATION

One bite: Calories 91; Fat 5g; (Sat 1.4g); Protein 3.4g; Carbs 9.3g; Fiber 1.5g; Sodium 36mg

Classic Avocado Toast

Makes 2 pieces

Avocado toast has become a bit of a culinary phenomenon recently. Packed with a wide variety of vitamins and minerals as well as healthy fats, avocado is the perfect snack for your baby. Plus, its rich, buttery texture makes it easy to spread on toast.

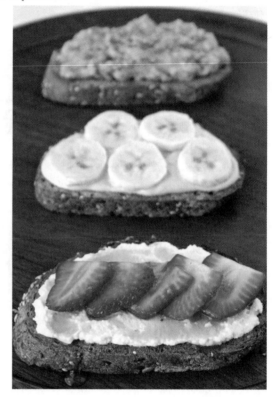

 I medium ripe Haas avocado
 I teaspoon fresh lemon juice
 2 slices toasted whole grain bread
 Kosher salt, to taste

Scoop the flesh out of the avocado with a spoon and place it in a bowl. Add the lemon juice and coarsely mash it with a fork.

Spread the avocado mixture on the toast and sprinkle a pinch of salt on top.

NUTRITIONAL INFORMATION

One piece: Calories 229; Fat 14.7g; (Sat 2.4g); Protein 5.5g; Carbs 20g; Fiber 8.7g; Sodium 116mg

Trendy Toast

Snacks don't have to be complicated. Simply toast some whole grain bread and slather on your tot's favorite toppings for a filling and nutritious snack. Try classic avocado toast or one of the other variations below. Or make your own creation—the possibilities are endless!

Creamy Almond with Banana Wheels

Makes 2 pieces

Your baby won't be able to resist this delectable treat that combines creamy yogurt with almond butter and banana slices. By giving snacks kid-friendly names like "banana wheels," it may make your children more excited to try them.

¼ cup vanilla Greek yogurt

1 tablespoon almond butter

2 slices toasted whole grain bread

½ banana, peeled and sliced

Mix the yogurt and almond butter together in a bowl until smooth. Spread the mixture on the toast and arrange the banana "wheels" on top.

NUTRITIONAL INFORMATION

One piece: Calories 169; Fat 5.9g; (Sat 1.2g); Protein 7g; Carbs 23.7g; Fiber 3.5g; Sodium 129mg

Ricotta, Strawberries and Honey

Makes 2 pieces

Creamy ricotta cheese is paired with juicy strawberries and a touch of honey in this easy, kid-friendly snack.

¼ cup ricotta cheese

⅛ teaspoon vanilla extract

2 slices toasted whole grain bread

4 strawberries, sliced

1 teaspoon honey

Mix the ricotta and vanilla together in a bowl. Spread the mixture on the toast and arrange the strawberries on top. Drizzle with honey and serve.

NUTRITIONAL INFORMATION

One piece: Calories 140; Fat 4.8g; (Sat 2.8g); Protein 7.1g; Carbs 17g; Fiber 2.4g; Sodium 134mg

Roasted Broccoli Pesto

Makes 2 cups

This recipe comes courtesy of Bev Weidner, the multi-talented food blogger from Bev Cooks (www. bevcooks.com) and mother to the most adorable, photogenic twins imaginable. This nutritious pesto gets rich depth of flavor from roasting the broccoli and garlic in the oven. It's a nice twist on classic pesto and is delicious served on toast or tossed with your favorite pasta.

4 cups broccoli florets (from 2 medium heads)
4 cloves garlic, in their skins
½ cup plus 2 tablespoons extra-virgin olive oil
2 tablespoons pine nuts, lightly toasted
¼ cup freshly grated Parmesan cheese
2 teaspoons fresh lemon juice
Toasted whole grain bread
Salt and pepper

Preheat oven to 400°F.

Place the broccoli florets and garlic on a baking sheet. Toss them with 2 tablespoons olive oil and season with a pinch of salt and pepper. Roast for 30 minutes, flipping them hallway through.

Transfer the broccoli and garlic (squeezed out of their skins) to a food processor. Add the pine nuts, cheese, and lemon juice, along with another small pinch of salt and pepper. With the motor running, add ½ cup olive oil in a thin stream until you get a smooth consistency.

Serve on toast or toss with pasta.

NUTRITIONAL INFORMATION

One piece toast plus 2 tablespoons pesto: Calories 166; Fat 10.2g; (Sat 1.7g); Protein 4.9g; Carbs 13.3g; Fiber 2.6g; Sodium 158mg

Avocado Yogurt Dip

Makes I cup

Creamy avocado and Greek yogurt join forces in this delectable dip, while lime juice and cumin add a flavor punch!

I medium ripe Haas avocado
¼ cup Greek yogurt
¼ teaspoon lime juice
⅛ teaspoon cumin
Salt and pepper, to taste

Puree all ingredients together in a food processor until smooth. Season with a pinch of salt and pepper.

NUTRITIONAL INFORMATION
One serving (¼ cup): Calories 91; Fat 7.2g (Sat 1.3g); Protein 2.5g; Carbs 4.9g; Fiber 3.4g; Sodium 80mg

Dynamite Dips

Toddlers love dipping food into sauces and spreads. Even picky eaters will eat healthy snacks when they're dipped into these tasty creations. Try serving these dips with fresh vegetables (like bell pepper strips, cucumber slices, and broccoli florets), fruit (like apple or banana slices), pretzels, or pieces of dry toast.

Creamy Pumpkin Dip

Makes I ½ cups

Pumpkin adds nutrients as well as a lovely orange color to this smooth and creamy treat that's delicious served with fresh fruit.

¼ cup vanilla Greek yogurt
2 ounces plain cream cheese, softened
I cup canned pumpkin puree
⅛ teaspoon cinnamon

Whisk the yogurt and cream cheese together in a bowl until smooth. Whisk in the pumpkin puree and cinnamon until well combined.

NUTRITIONAL INFORMATION
One serving (¼ cup): Calories 54; Fat 3g (Sat 2g); Protein 1.5g; Carbs 5.1g; Fiber 1.2g; Sodium 38mg

Classic Hummus

Makes 1½ cups

It's easy to make your own hummus at home. Rich in flavor and nutrients, hummus is perfect for dipping fresh vegetables, pretzels, pieces of toast, or rice cakes. It's also delicious when spread on sandwiches (see Turkey and Hummus Pinwheels on page 206). Throw some roasted red peppers or steamed spinach into the food processor for delicious variations of this base recipe.

1 can (15 ounces) reduced-sodium chickpeas, rinsed and drained
½ clove garlic
2 tablespoons tahini*
2 tablespoons fresh lemon juice

¼ teaspoon ground cumin
1½ tablespoons olive oil
3 tablespoons water
Salt and pepper, to taste

Place the chickpeas, garlic, tahini, lemon juice, and cumin together in a food processor and pulse until finely chopped. With the motor running, pour in the olive oil. Add the water and continue to blend until smooth. Season with a pinch of salt and pepper.

*Tahini is a paste made from ground sesame seeds and can be found in specialty grocery stores.

NUTRITIONAL INFORMATION

One serving (¼ cup): Calories 146; Fat 6.5g (Sat 0.9g); Protein 4.5g; Carbs 17.9g; Fiber 3.5g; Sodium 213mg

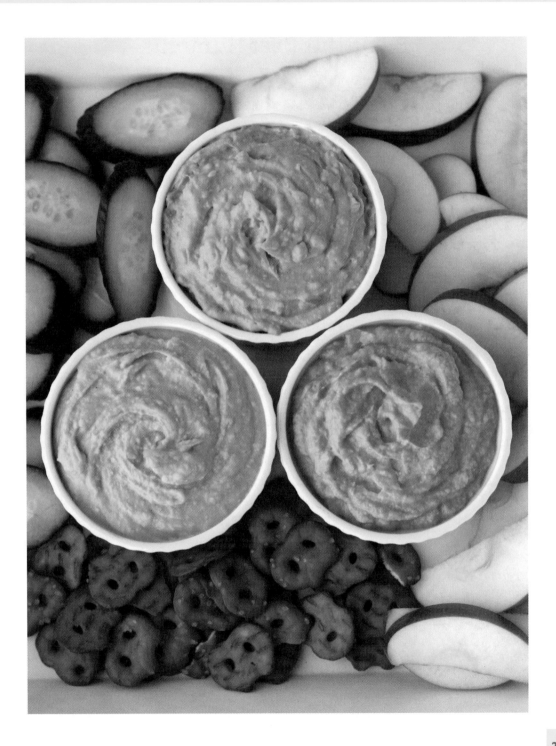

Beautiful Beet Hummus

Makes about 2 cups

This recipe was shared by the talented Katie Mor-ford from the site Mom's Kitchen Handbook (www.momskitchenhandbook.com). Her spin on classic hummus uses nutritious beets, which give the dish a rich flavor and vibrant, ruby color. As Katie suggests, you can save time by buying pre-cooked beets in vacuum-sealed pouches in some grocery stores. This also makes an excellent canapé for adults, served on chilled cucumber slices and topped with fresh goat cheese.

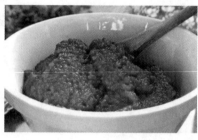

3 large red beets, cooked and peeled*
2 to 3 tablespoons water
½ cup roasted almonds
3 tablespoons extra-virgin olive oil

2 tablespoons fresh lemon juice
1 small clove garlic, peeled
Salt, to taste

Cut the beets into quarters and put them into the bowl of a food processor. Add one tablespoon water, the almonds, olive oil, lemon juice, garlic, and a pinch of salt. Puree until smooth. Add another tablespoon or two of water as needed to thin the hummus to desired consistency. Taste, and add a little more salt if needed.

To serve as an appetizer, spoon about 1½ teaspoons of Beet Hummus onto a slice of chilled, unpeeled English cucumber. Top with a dot of fresh goat cheese.

*See Beet Puree recipe (page 99) for directions on how to cook beets.

NUTRITIONAL INFORMATION

One serving (¼ cup): Calories 110; Fat 9.2g (Sat 1.1g); Protein 2.4g; Carbs 5.2g; Fiber 1.8g; Sodium 60mg

Very Berry Smoothie

Makes 2 smoothies

This berry-licious smoothie is packed with vitamin C, antioxidants, protein, and more. Ground flaxseed adds a boost of omega-3 fatty acids and health-promoting phytochemicals.

1 ½ cups mixed berries like blueberries, strawberries, blackberries, and raspberries

1 banana, peeled

½ cup vanilla Greek yogurt

¼ cup milk

1 tablespoon ground flaxseed or chia seeds

Ice

Blend all ingredients in a blender until smooth. Pour into two glasses and serve.

NUTRITIONAL INFORMATION

One serving: Calories 184; Fat 4.8g (Sat 2.2g); Protein 6.4g; Carbs 34.3g; Fiber 7.1g; Sodium 56mg

Flaxseed

Flaxseeds are an excellent addition to your baby's diet. Rich in fiber, omega-3 fatty acids, and phytochemicals (plant-based compounds) called lignans, which have several health benefits, ground flaxseed is absorbed well by the body, as opposed to whole flaxseeds, which are difficult to digest and pass through the body without giving much nutritional benefit. Purchase ground flaxseed, or else purchase whole flaxseed and grind it in a blender or spice grinder as needed. Sprinkle it on yogurt or oatmeal or add it to smoothies, sauces, and pancake or muffin batter. You can store unused flaxseed in a cool, dry place or in the refrigerator.

Tropical Green Smoothie

Makes 2 smoothies

Your baby will enjoy a taste of the tropics in this vibrant, green smoothie that combines spinach with naturally sweet fruit and creamy coconut milk.

1 cup packed baby spinach

1 cup chopped pineapple

1 banana

¾ cup coconut milk

Ice

Blend all ingredients in a blender until smooth. Pour into two glasses and serve.

NUTRITIONAL INFORMATION

One serving: Calories 263; Fat 17.2g (Sat 16.1g); Protein 3.2g; Carbs 27.2g; Fiber 3g; Sodium 23mg

Smoothie Party!

Smoothies are a great way to expose your little one to a wide variety of fruits, and even vegetables. They will come in handy when your baby becomes a toddler and may not be as willing to try new foods. You can mix in all sorts of nutritious ingredients, like flaxseed, chia seeds, Greek yogurt, oats, and more. Frozen fruit like berries, peaches, and pineapple are perfect for smoothies—you can toss them into the blender straight from the freezer. If using fresh fruit, you can add a few ice cubes to the blender to make your smoothies nice and frothy.

Peanut Butter Banana Smoothie

Makes 2 smoothies

This yummy treat has plenty of protein and calcium as well as a boost of nutritious whole grains from oats.

¾ cup vanilla Greek yogurt
½ cup milk
1 banana

2 tablespoons peanut butter
⅓ cup old-fashioned oats
Ice

Blend all ingredients in a blender until smooth. Pour into two glasses and serve.

NUTRITIONAL INFORMATION

One serving: Calories 331; Fat 12.3g (Sat 4.1g); Protein 14.4g; Carbs 43.1g; Fiber 4.3g; Sodium 163mg

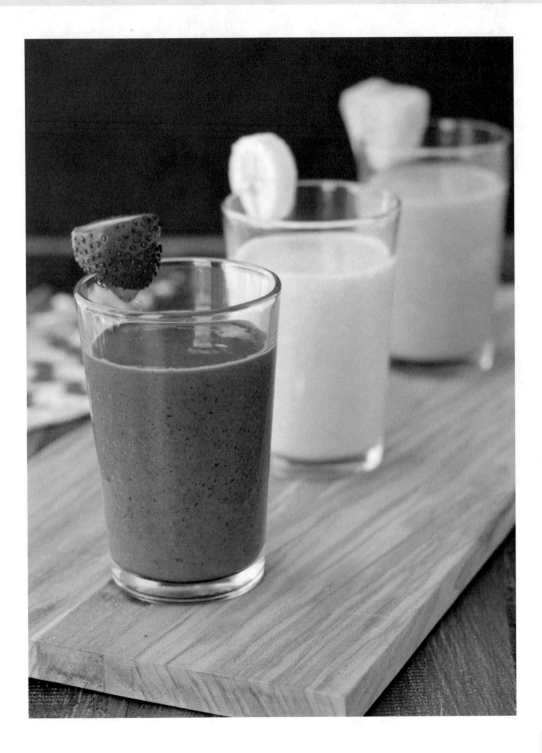

Parsnip Pear Soup,
page 223

Soups

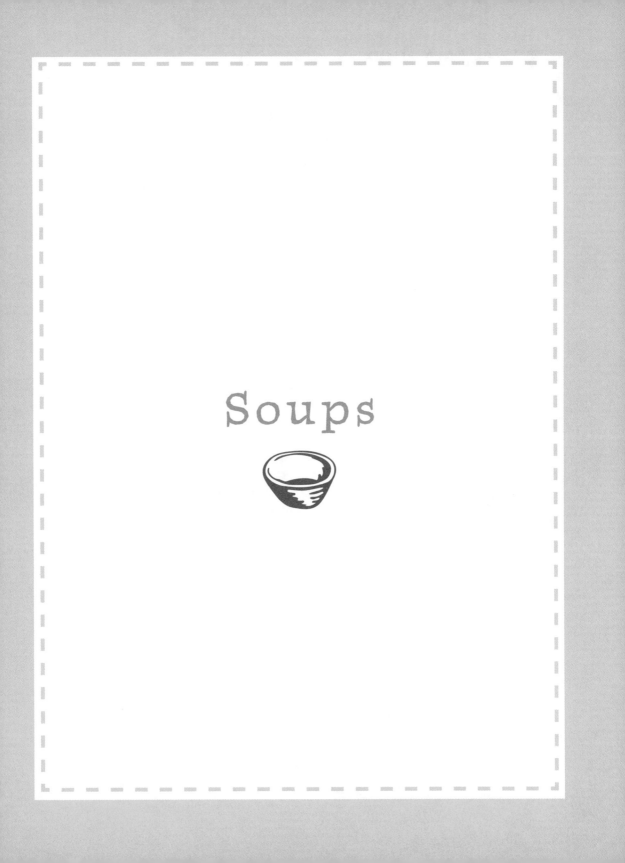

Pasta Fagioli

Makes 8 servings

Pasta fagioli is a classic Italian soup with humble peasant origins. Made from inexpensive ingredients like pasta and beans, it's a comforting, stick-to-your-ribs dish that's satisfying and full of flavor.

1 tablespoon olive oil
2 ounces pancetta, diced (optional)
1 medium yellow onion, diced
2 large carrots, peeled and diced
2 stalks celery, diced
3 cloves garlic, minced
1½ teaspoons chopped, fresh rosemary
 or ½ teaspoon dried
1 bay leaf
1 can (14.5 ounces) crushed tomatoes

2 quarts low-sodium chicken or
 vegetable broth
2 cans (15.5 oz) low-sodium cannellini
 beans, drained and rinsed
1½ cups small pasta like ditalini or elbows
 (preferably whole grain)
2 tablespoons grated Parmigiano-Reggiano
 cheese plus extra for garnish
Salt and pepper, to taste

Heat the oil in a large Dutch oven or other heavy-bottomed pot over medium heat. Add the pancetta (if using) and cook a couple of minutes until it starts to brown. Add the onion, carrots, and celery and cook, stirring occasionally, until partially softened, 5–6 minutes. Add the garlic, rosemary, and bay leaf and cook another minute until fragrant. Add the tomatoes and chicken broth and raise the heat to bring it to a simmer.

Place about a quarter cup of beans in a bowl and add a little bit of the cooking liquid. Mash them together to form a paste and add it to the pot along with the rest of the whole beans. Cover the pot and simmer the soup for 15 minutes. Add the pasta and simmer another 15 minutes, uncovered, until pasta is tender. Stir in the cheese.

Taste the soup and season with pinch each of salt and pepper. Ladle the soup into bowls and top with extra grated cheese, if desired. Soup will thicken as it stands.

NUTRITIONAL INFORMATION
One serving: Calories 267; Fat 4.6g (Sat 1.2g); Protein 16.4g; Carbs 42.2g; Fiber 8.5g; Sodium 481mg

Parsnip Pear Soup

Makes 8 servings

This recipe was shared by my talented friend Jessica Fishman Levinson, founder of the nutrition site Nutritioulicious (www.nutritioulicious.com). Jessica is a big fan of soup, especially hot, comforting bowls of soup that warm you up from the inside out. This dish definitely fits the bill. Parsnips give the soup a velvety, creamy texture without any cream. Pears and a touch of maple syrup add a hint of sweetness. This delicious soup is equally suitable for a casual weeknight meal or a festive holiday dinner.

1 tablespoon olive oil
½ cup diced shallots
1 garlic clove, minced
1½ pounds parsnips, peeled and diced
3 cups diced pears (about 1 pound)
6 cups low-sodium vegetable broth

2 sprigs thyme
2 tablespoons pure maple syrup
1 tablespoon white wine vinegar
¼ teaspoon kosher salt
Freshly ground pepper, to taste

Heat the oil in a large soup pot over medium heat. Add the shallots and garlic and sauté 1–2 minutes until slightly softened. Stir in the parsnips and cook for 2 minutes. Cover the pot and cook another 5 minutes until the parsnips are tender and starting to brown. Stir in the pears. Cover and cook another 5 minutes.

Add the broth and thyme. Bring to a boil, and then reduce heat to a simmer and cook, uncovered, for 30 minutes.

Remove the pot from the heat and remove the thyme stems. Using an immersion blender, carefully puree the soup until smooth. Stir in the maple syrup, vinegar, salt, and pepper.

NUTRITIONAL INFORMATION

One serving (one generous cup): Calories 143; Fat 2g (Sat 0.3g); Protein 1.5g; Carbs 31g; Fiber 7g; Sodium 176mg

Turkey Florentine
Meatballs, page 228

Dinner

Pretzel-Crusted Chicken Tenders with Honey Mustard Dipping Sauce

Makes 4 servings

Are you looking for a fun new way to serve chicken? These chicken tenders are coated in crushed pretzels and baked in the oven to crispy perfection. Serve them with my honey mustard dipping sauce for the perfect kid- and adult-friendly dish!

¼ cup flour
2 eggs
1½ cups crushed pretzels*
1 pound chicken tenders

¼ teaspoon salt
⅛ teaspoon pepper
Olive oil

Honey Mustard Dipping Sauce:
¼ cup Dijon mustard
¼ cup honey
¼ cup plain Greek yogurt

Preheat oven to 400°F. Spray or brush a baking sheet generously with olive oil.

To make the honey mustard dipping sauce, mix the mustard, honey, and yogurt together in a medium bowl.

Prepare your breading station. Place the flour in a shallow dish. Mix the eggs with 2 tablespoons water in a second dish. Place the crushed pretzels in a third dish.

Season the chicken with salt and pepper. Dip each chicken tender into the flour, shaking off any excess. Then dip into the egg and finally the pretzel crumbs, coating all sides well.

Place the chicken tenders on the prepared baking sheet and spray or brush them with olive oil. Bake in the oven for 8 minutes, and then flip and bake another 6–8 until chicken is cooked through.

Serve chicken tenders with honey mustard dipping sauce.

NUTRITIONAL INFORMATION

One serving chicken: Calories 290; Fat 5.1g (Sat 1.6g); Protein 30.3g; Carbs 26.4g; Fiber 0.9g; Sodium 385mg

---

NUTRITIONAL INFORMATION

One serving (2 tablespoons) sauce: Calories 69; Fat 1.3g (Sat 0.2g); Protein 0.6g; Carbs 12.4g; Fiber 0g; Sodium 257mg

*To crush the pretzels, place them in a food processor and process until they're mostly fine crumbs with some larger crumbs. Alternatively, you can put them in a sealed plastic bag and crush them with a rolling pin.

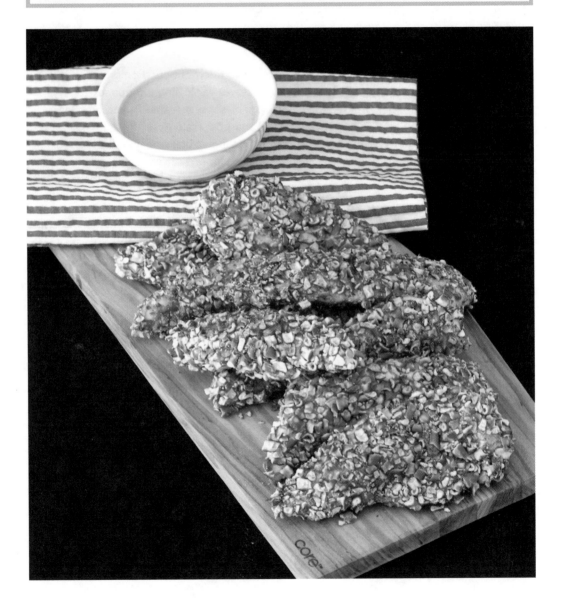

Turkey Florentine Meatballs

Makes about 26 meatballs

These adorable meatballs are packed with flavor and nutrients. Spinach adds a wide variety of important vitamins and minerals, including vitamin K, vitamin A, folate, iron, and calcium. Bake them in the oven for a quick and healthy meal that the whole family will love. Serve them with Veggie-Packed Tomato Sauce (page 229) or your favorite jarred tomato sauce.

2 ounces whole wheat bread (about 2 slices), torn into pieces
⅓ cup milk
5 ounces frozen chopped spinach (or fresh spinach, steamed and chopped)
1 package (1.2 pounds) 93 percent lean ground turkey
1 large egg
⅓ cup finely chopped onion
2 cloves garlic, finely chopped
6 tablespoons grated Parmesan cheese
1 teaspoon salt
¼ teaspoon black pepper
2 tablespoons olive oil
Veggie-Packed Tomato Sauce (page 229) or marinara sauce for serving

Preheat oven to 375°F. Line a baking sheet with parchment paper.

Place the bread and milk in a small bowl and let it soak.

Defrost the spinach according to package directions. Squeeze the water out of the spinach and place it in a large bowl. Add the turkey, egg, onion, garlic, cheese, salt and pepper. Add the milk-soaked bread and mix all of the ingredients together.

Form the mixture into small meatballs, about 1½ tablespoons each. Place the meatballs on the prepared baking sheet and brush them with olive oil.

Bake in the oven 20–25 minutes until cooked through. Toss the meatballs with your favorite tomato sauce.

NUTRITIONAL INFORMATION

One meatball: Calories 58; Fat 3.3g (Sat 1g); Protein 5.2g; Carbs 1.7g; Fiber 0.3g; Sodium 117mg

Veggie-Packed Tomato Sauce

Makes about 4 cups

This all-purpose tomato sauce is packed with tons of healthy vegetables! Don't worry about chopping the vegetables perfectly, since you will be pureeing it all in the end anyway. For faster prep, chop the veggies in a food processor. Serve this sauce with Turkey Florentine Meatballs (page 228), Zucchini Tots (page 198), Crispy Tofu Nuggets (page 200) or Cauliflower Cheesy Bread (202).

2 tablespoons olive oil
1 medium yellow onion, chopped
1 medium carrot, peeled and chopped
1 medium zucchini, chopped
½ red bell pepper, chopped
2 cloves garlic, chopped
1 can (28 ounces) crushed tomatoes
1 bay leaf
1 teaspoon dried Italian seasoning (or a
    mixture of dried basil, oregano, and
    thyme)
¾ teaspoon kosher salt
¼ teaspoon black pepper

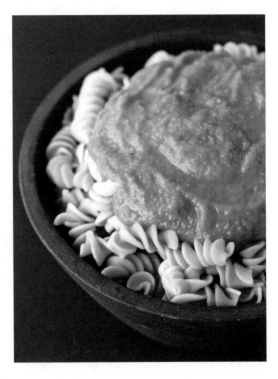

Heat the oil in a large saucepan over medium-high heat and add the onion, carrot, zucchini, bell pepper, and garlic. Cook, stirring occasionally, until vegetables start to soften, 6–7 minutes. Stir in the crushed tomatoes, bay leaf, Italian seasoning, salt, and pepper. Cover and simmer on medium-low heat until vegetables are tender, 25–30 minutes.

Remove the bay leaf and carefully puree the sauce with an immersion blender until smooth (or leave it slightly chunky for more texture). The sauce will be thick, so add water as needed to thin it out to desired consistency. Sauce can be stored in the refrigerator or frozen for later use.

NUTRITIONAL INFORMATION

One serving (½ cup): Calories 71; Fat 3.2g (Sat 0.5g); Protein 2.1g; Carbs 10.2g; Fiber 2.7g; Sodium 252mg

Chicken, Broccoli, and Rice Skillet Bake

Makes 6 servings

Casseroles like this can be a lifesaver on busy nights. Just start cooking your ingredients in a skillet and then transfer it to the oven to finish cooking. This family-friendly dish is a well-balanced meal and contains protein, vegetables, and whole grains. Traditional casseroles often use canned soup, which can be very high in sodium. Make this dish instead, using fresh, wholesome ingredients. You can use frozen brown rice—it's a great time saver.

3 cups broccoli florets, fresh or frozen
2 tablespoons olive oil
1 pound chicken breast, cut into bite-sized pieces
¼ teaspoon salt
⅛ teaspoon black pepper
½ teaspoon dried Italian seasoning or thyme
1 small yellow onion, finely chopped

2 cloves garlic, minced
2 tablespoons flour
1 cup low-sodium chicken broth
¾ cup milk
1 tablespoon Dijon mustard
⅓ cup plain Greek yogurt
1¼ cups shredded cheddar cheese, divided use
3 cups cooked brown rice

Preheat oven to 375° F.

Steam the broccoli in a steamer basket for a few minutes, until crisp-tender.

Heat ½ tablespoon oil in a large oven-safe skillet (preferably cast iron) over medium-high heat and add the chicken. Season the chicken with salt, pepper, and Italian seasoning. Cook 3 minutes until browned, then flip and cook another 2–3 minutes. Remove chicken from skillet.

Heat the remaining 1½ tablespoons oil in the skillet and add the onion and garlic. Sauté a few minutes until softened. Add the flour and stir to combine. Whisk in the chicken broth, milk, and mustard. Simmer a few minutes until sauce thickens. Remove from heat and whisk in the yogurt and 1 cup of cheese.

Add the cooked rice, broccoli, and chicken (along with any juices) to the skillet and stir to combine. Sprinkle the remaining ¼ cup cheese on top and transfer the skillet to the oven. Bake for 20–25 minutes until cheese is melted and casserole is bubbly. Let cool slightly and serve.

NUTRITIONAL INFORMATION

One serving: Calories 399; Fat 15.7g (Sat 7.1g); Protein 28.4g; Carbs 32.6g; Fiber 3.3g; Sodium 445mg

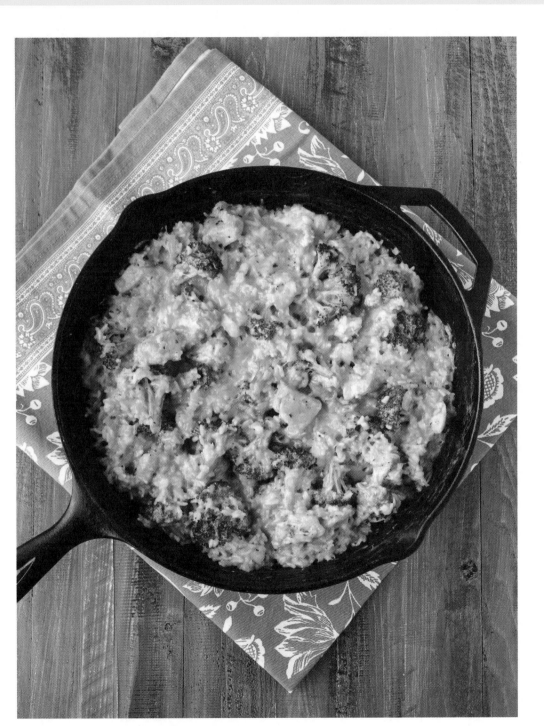

Creamy Chicken and Corn Taquitos

Makes 12 taquitos

A taquito is a Mexican snack consisting of a rolled-up tortilla, which is stuffed with fillings like meat, beans, or cheese, and then fried. Taquitos are the perfect kid-friendly food. You can stuff them with whatever nutritious ingredients you like and they're also easy to pick up and dip into sauces. Unlike traditional taquitos (which are deep fried) mine are baked in the oven, making them much healthier. Instead of corn, you can substitute other ingredients like spinach or black beans. Use rotisserie chicken from the grocery store to save time.

3 ounces cream cheese, softened
¼ cup mild green (tomatillo) salsa
1 teaspoon cumin
¼ teaspoon garlic powder
2 cups shredded, cooked chicken
3 ounces (about 1 cup) shredded
   Monterey Jack or Mexican blend
   cheese
½ cup cooked corn
12 small (6-inch) flour tortillas
Olive oil

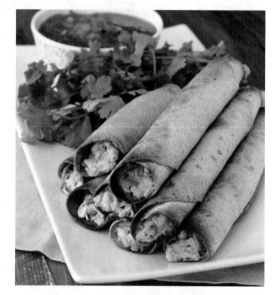

Preheat oven to 400°F. Brush or spray a baking sheet with olive oil.

Mix the cream cheese, salsa, cumin, and garlic powder together in a bowl. Stir in the chicken, cheese and corn.

Place each tortilla on a cutting board. Spoon about 2–3 tablespoons of the filling on the lower third of the tortilla, keeping the filling about 1 inch from the edges. Roll the tortillas up as tightly as you can. Place them seam side down on the baking sheet. Brush the tops and side of the taquitos with olive oil or spray with olive oil cooking spray.

Bake in the oven until crispy and golden brown, about 15 minutes. Remove from oven and let cool slightly before serving. Serve taquitos with your favorite dipping sauce or Avocado Yogurt Dip (page 213).

NUTRITIONAL INFORMATION

One taquito: Calories 222; Fat 6.8g (Sat 3.3g); Protein 13.4g; Carbs 24.3g; Fiber 0.6g; Sodium 345mg

Pasta with Creamy Tomato Sauce and Chicken Sausage

Makes 8 servings

This family-friendly pasta dish has all of the flavors of lasagna with none of the fuss. The sauce couldn't be simpler—just simmer tomatoes with some aromatics in a saucepan and then stir in creamy ricotta cheese and Parmesan. I like to use strained tomatoes or tomato puree (also known as passata) because it gives a nice, smooth sauce with a mild flavor. If you can't find it, you can use crushed tomatoes, which have a chunkier texture and more assertive tomato flavor.

1 carton (26 ounces) strained tomatoes or tomato puree like Pomi brand
3 tablespoons olive oil, divided use
1 clove garlic, smashed
½ teaspoon kosher salt
¼ teaspoon sugar
1 sprig basil

1 pound penne, mezze rigatoni, or other pasta
1 package (12 oz) cooked chicken sausage like Aidells Italian Style
1 cup ricotta cheese
¼ cup grated Parmesan cheese plus extra for topping

Place the tomatoes, 2 tablespoons olive oil, garlic, salt, sugar, and basil together in a saucepan and simmer, covered, for 20 minutes. Discard the garlic and basil.

Meanwhile, cook the pasta according to package directions. Drain.

Cut the sausage into small (¼-inch) pieces. Heat the remaining 1 tablespoon olive oil in a large skillet over medium-high heat and brown the sausage. Lower the heat and add the tomato sauce, pasta, ricotta, and Parmesan cheeses. Stir until ingredients are combined and sauce is smooth and creamy. Serve with extra Parmesan cheese on the side.

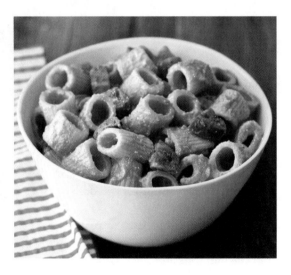

NUTRITIONAL INFORMATION

One serving: Calories 428; Fat 16.1g (Sat 5.7g); Protein 19.8g; Carbs 49.2g; Fiber 3.3g; Sodium 516mg

Chicken Parmesan Sliders

Makes 8 sliders

These mini chicken burgers are sure to be a hit with your family. They combine two classic favorites—burgers and chicken Parmesan. And their small size makes them more appealing to young eaters. They're packed with protein, fiber, and zinc, and also supply a good amount of iron and calcium.

I pound ground chicken or turkey
I clove garlic, minced
¾ cup lower-sodium marinara sauce, divided use
I ounce (about ¼ cup) grated Parmesan cheese

½ teaspoon dried oregano or thyme
¼ teaspoon kosher salt
I tablespoon olive oil
¾ cup shredded mozzarella cheese
8 whole grain slider buns, toasted
Handful of fresh basil leaves, chopped

Mix the chicken, garlic, ¼ cup marinara sauce, Parmesan cheese, oregano (or thyme), and salt together in a large bowl. Form into 8 small (½-inch thick) patties. Wet your hand with a small amount of water if the patties stick to your hands.

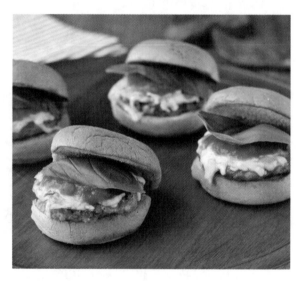

Heat the oil in a large nonstick skillet over medium high heat and add the patties. Cook for 4–5 minutes, then flip and cook for another 4 minutes, or until completely cooked through. During the last minute of cooking, add about 1½ tablespoons cheese on top of each burger and cover the skillet to melt the cheese.

To serve, place the cooked patties on toasted slider buns. Top each patty with a tablespoon of marinara sauce and some basil. Add the bun tops and serve with extra marinara sauce on the side.

NUTRITIONAL INFORMATION

One slider: Calories 242; Fat 7.8g (Sat 3g); Protein 19.3g; Carbs 22g; Fiber 3.4g; Sodium 407mg

Turkey Sloppy Joes

Makes 5 sandwiches

Kids and adults will love this classic sandwich. Skip the canned version and make your own sloppy Joes at home—they're more nutritious and they'll taste a whole lot better. I add kidney beans to the mix for extra texture as well as a boost of protein, vitamins, and minerals. Don't worry if you make a mess while eating it—that's half the fun!

1 tablespoon olive oil
1 small yellow onion, finely chopped
1 carrot, peeled and grated
2 cloves garlic, finely chopped
1 pound ground turkey or lean ground beef
¼ cup tomato paste
1 cup low-sodium canned kidney beans, drained and rinsed

1½ cups canned tomato sauce (no salt added)
1 tablespoon Worcestershire sauce
1½ tablespoons molasses or brown sugar
2 teaspoons cider vinegar
5 whole wheat rolls, for serving
Kosher salt and black pepper, to taste

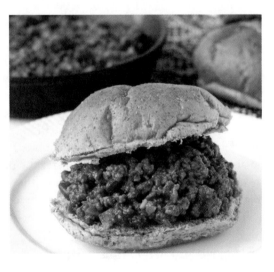

Heat the oil in a large skillet over medium high heat. Add the onion, carrot, and garlic and cook for 4–5 minutes until they start to soften. Add the turkey and season it with a pinch of salt and pepper. Brown the turkey, breaking it up with a spatula as it cooks. Once turkey is browned, stir in the tomato paste, and cook another 1–2 minutes. Stir in the beans, tomato sauce, Worcestershire sauce, molasses, vinegar, ¾ teaspoon salt, and ¼ teaspoon pepper.

Simmer on medium-low heat for 10–15 minutes until turkey is cooked and sauce is thickened. Serve on whole wheat rolls.

NUTRITIONAL INFORMATION

One serving (filling only): Calories 282; Fat 9.9g (Sat 2.4g); Protein 21.7g; Carbs 26.4g; Fiber 4.7g; Sodium 572mg

Sunday Beef Stew

Makes 6-8 servings

This stew is a comforting, stick-to-your-ribs dish that's perfect for those lazy Sunday afternoons when you just don't feel like leaving the house. Once all of the ingredients are seared in the pot, simply throw it in the oven and in a few hours, you'll have a delicious and hearty meal that the whole family will love. Beef is a rich source of protein, iron, vitamin B12, and zinc.

2½ pounds boneless beef chuck, trimmed of fat and cut into 1 ½-inch pieces
½ teaspoon salt
¼ teaspoon pepper
2 tablespoons olive oil, divided use
1 large yellow onion, chopped
4 cloves garlic, chopped
2 tablespoons tomato paste
2 tablespoons flour

3 cups reduced-sodium beef stock
2 sprigs fresh thyme (or ½ teaspoon dried)
1 bay leaf
12 ounces peeled baby rainbow carrots or 3 cups carrots sliced into 1-inch pieces
1 pound small Yukon gold or red potatoes, washed and cut in half
¼ cup fresh, chopped parsley (optional)

Preheat oven to 325°F.

Season the beef with salt and pepper. Heat 1 tablespoon oil in a Dutch oven or large pot over medium-high heat. Add half of the beef to the hot oil and sear it on all sides until browned, 5–6 minutes. Transfer the meat to a plate. Repeat with the remaining oil and beef.

Add the onion and garlic to the pot and cook a few minutes until softened. Stir in the tomato paste. Add the beef and its juices back to the pot and sprinkle with flour. Stir until flour is dissolved, 1–2 minutes. Add the beef stock, thyme, and bay leaf, and stir with a wooden spoon to scrape up any brown bits from the bottom of the pot. Bring the mixture to a simmer and cover the pot. Transfer the pot to the oven.

Bake for 2 hours, and then remove the pot from the oven and stir in the carrots and potatoes. Cover and return the pot to the oven for another hour until the vegetables are cooked through. Adjust seasoning to taste. Stir in the parsley and serve.

NUTRITIONAL INFORMATION

One serving (⅛ of the dish): Calories 291; Fat 10.1g (Sat 3.3g); Protein 33.4g; Carbs 18.2g; Fiber 3.3g; Sodium 389mg

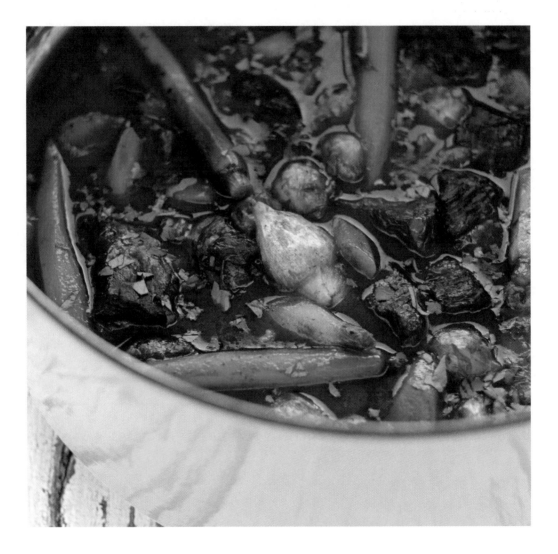

Barbecue Cheddar Mini Meatloaves

Makes 4 mini meatloaves

These kid-sized meatloaves are flavored with barbecue sauce and studded with yummy cheddar cheese. Barbecue sauce is popular with children because of its sweet and tangy flavor. Many store-bought varieties can have very large amounts of sugar, so read the labels and try to find a brand that has less sugar. Be sure to let the meatloaves cool slightly before serving, so that the cheese isn't too hot for little mouths!

I pound lean ground beef
¼ medium yellow onion, finely chopped
I large egg
6 tablespoons organic barbecue sauce, divided use
¼ cup quick-cooking oats* or panko breadcrumbs

¼ teaspoon salt
¼ teaspoon black pepper
½ cup (2 ounces) small-diced cheddar cheese

Preheat oven to 400°F.

Place the ground beef, onion, egg, 2 tablespoons barbecue sauce, oats, pepper, and cheese together in a large bowl and mix until combined.

Line a baking sheet with parchment paper or aluminum foil. Divide the mixture into four equal portions and form them into loaves on the baking sheet. Brush each meatloaf with 1 tablespoon barbecue sauce.

Bake 22–25 minutes until cooked through. Cool meatloaves slightly before serving.

*If you don't have quick-cooking oats, you can make them by pulsing old-fashioned oats in a food processor until coarsely ground.

NUTRITIONAL INFORMATION

One meatloaf: Calories 303; Fat 14g (Sat 6.5g); Protein 29.2g; Carbs 12.9g; Fiber 0.8g; Sodium 375mg

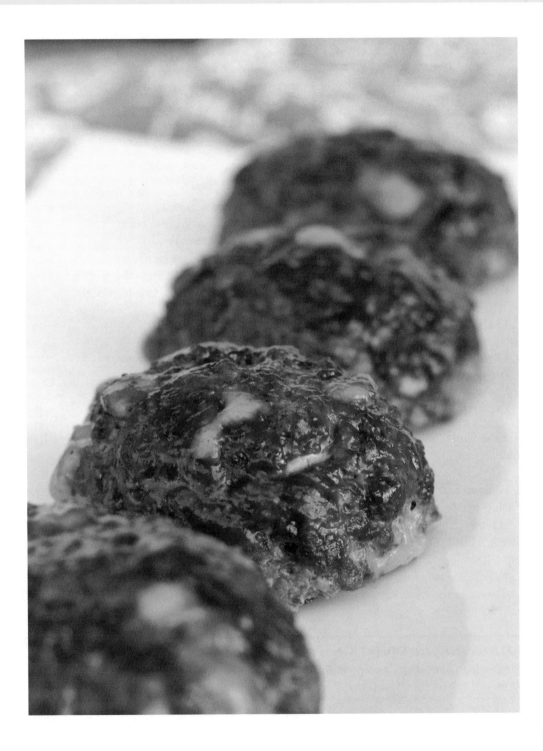

Lamb Kofta Kebabs with Tzatziki Sauce

Makes 12 kebabs or 4 servings

This is a meal that the whole family will enjoy! Kofta kebabs are made with ground meat rather than cubed meat, which makes it easier for your little ones to eat. Let them have fun dipping the kebabs in the yogurt sauce—just be sure to remove them from the skewers first. Lamb is an excellent source of iron and zinc for your baby.

Kebabs

1 pound ground lamb (or beef)
2 tablespoons grated or minced onion
2 cloves garlic, grated or minced
2 tablespoons chopped parsley
1½ teaspoons ground coriander

1 teaspoon ground cumin
¾ teaspoon salt
¼ teaspoon pepper
Olive oil, for brushing the grill
Flat bread, for serving (optional)

Tzatziki Sauce

1 cup plain whole milk Greek yogurt
½ cup grated cucumber, squeezed dry
1 small clove garlic, grated or minced
1 teaspoon lemon juice

1 teaspoon fresh mint or dill (or ¼
   teaspoon dried)
Pinch of salt

Mix the lamb, onion, garlic, parsley, coriander, cumin, salt, and pepper together in a large bowl.

Divide the mixture into 12 roughly even balls. Mold each ball around the pointed end of a skewer, making an oval kebab that comes to a point just covering the tip of the skewer. If using wooden skewers, soak them in water for 15 minutes before threading them.

Heat a grill pan over medium high heat or prepare a grill. Brush the pan lightly with olive oil. Grill the kebabs, turning occasionally, until brown all over and cooked through, about 10 minutes. Transfer to a serving platter and serve with tzatziki sauce and flat bread. Remove skewers before serving kebabs to your baby.

To make the tzatziki sauce, mix all of ingredients together in a bowl. Refrigerate until ready to serve.

NUTRITIONAL INFORMATION
One serving (3 kebabs): Calories 268; Fat 18.2g (Sat 9.3g); Protein 20.6g; Carbs 1.8g; Fiber 0.6g; Sodium 521mg

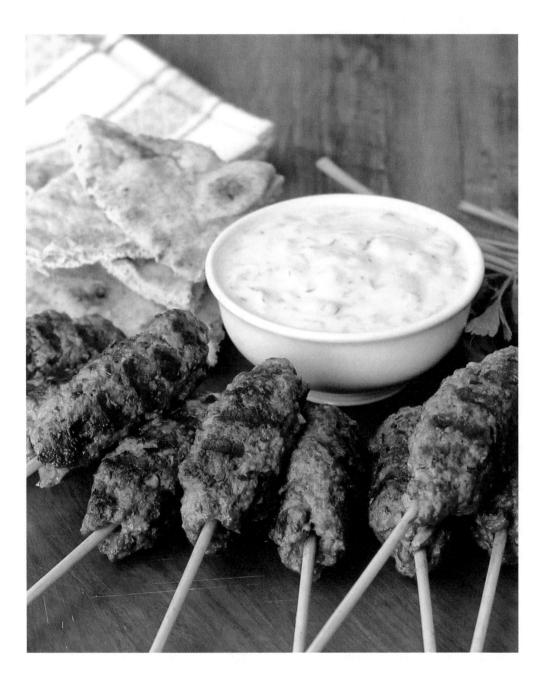

Pork and Vegetable Stir-Fry

Makes 4 servings

This healthy stir-fry uses pork tenderloin—a lean, tender cut of meat that has higher levels of vitamin B12, zinc and selenium when compared to chicken breast. The pork is cooked with fresh green beans, red bell peppers and mushrooms, but you can use any combination of vegetables that you like. To save time (and dishes), you can steam the green beans directly in the wok first. Stir fries cook quickly, so be sure to prep all of your ingredients before you start cooking.

3 tablespoons low-sodium soy sauce, divided use

3 teaspoons cornstarch, divided use

1 teaspoon sesame oil

1¼ teaspoons sugar, divided use

¾ pound pork tenderloin, thinly sliced

¼ cup low-sodium chicken broth

½ pound fresh green beans, trimmed and cut into 2-inch pieces

2 tablespoons peanut oil or other neutral flavored oil, divided use

2 teaspoons minced garlic

2 teaspoons minced ginger

1 red bell pepper, thinly sliced

4 ounces mushrooms, sliced

Black pepper, to taste

Brown rice for serving

To make the pork marinade, mix 1 tablespoon soy sauce, 1 teaspoon cornstarch, sesame oil, and ¼ teaspoon sugar together in a medium bowl. Add the pork and stir to coat all of the pieces with the marinade. Cover and set aside while you prepare the rest of the ingredients.

To make the sauce, stir the remaining 2 tablespoons soy sauce, 2 teaspoons cornstarch, 1 teaspoon sugar, and chicken broth together in a small bowl and set aside.

Heat a large wok or sauté pan over high heat and add the green beans and 2 tablespoons water. Cover the wok and steam the beans until crisp-tender, about 5 minutes. Remove the beans and dry the wok.

Heat 1 tablespoon peanut oil in the wok and add the pork. Cook the pork, stirring occasionally, 3–4 minutes until just cooked through. Remove the pork from the wok.

Heat the remaining 1 tablespoon peanut oil in the wok and add the garlic and ginger. Add the peppers and mushrooms and cook, stirring often, 3–4 minutes. Stir in the steamed green beans and cook another 2–3 minutes until tender. Add the pork to the wok along with any juices. Stir the sauce to distribute the cornstarch and add it to the skillet. Cook another few minutes until sauce thickens and pork is cooked through. Season with black pepper to taste. Serve stir-fry with brown rice.

NUTRITIONAL INFORMATION

One serving: Calories 215; Fat 9.3g (Sat 2g); Protein 20.6g; Carbs 11.7g; Fiber 2.6g; Sodium 616mg

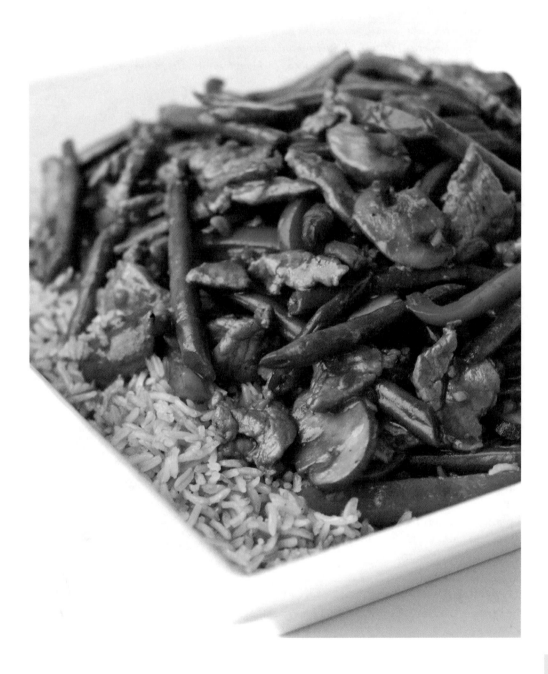

Salmon Cakes with Dilly Yogurt

Makes 4 servings

These moist, petite cakes are a great way to get your children to eat salmon, which is one of the richest sources of omega-3 fatty acids. Their small size also makes them a great finger food for young eaters. You can also make larger cakes and serve them on buns as salmon burgers.

Dilly Yogurt
½ cup plain Greek yogurt
1 teaspoon Dijon mustard

2 teaspoons chopped dill
1 teaspoon lemon juice

Salmon Cakes
1 pound salmon fillets, skin removed and cut into chunks
2 tablespoons sliced scallions
1 tablespoon mayonnaise
1 teaspoon Dijon mustard
1 teaspoon lemon juice

¼ cup panko breadcrumbs, preferably whole wheat
½ teaspoon salt
¼ teaspoon black pepper
1 tablespoon olive oil, for frying

To make the Dilly Yogurt, mix the yogurt, mustard, dill, and lemon juice together in a small bowl. Refrigerate until ready to use.

Pulse the salmon in a food processor until finely chopped. Transfer to a bowl and add the scallions, mayonnaise, mustard, lemon juice, breadcrumbs, salt, and pepper. Mix until combined. Form the mixture into eight small cakes.

Heat the oil in a large skillet over medium heat. Add the salmon cakes and cook 2–3 minutes until golden brown. Flip and cook another 2–3 minutes on the second side. Remove from pan and serve with Dilly Yogurt.

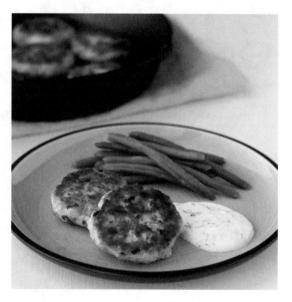

NUTRITIONAL INFORMATION
One serving: Calories 308; Fat 15.5g (Sat 3.3g); Protein 25g; Carbs 5.7g; Fiber 0.5g; Sodium 453mg

Tilapia Oreganata

Makes 4 servings

A simple topping of breadcrumbs, herbs, lemon, and olive oil is the perfect way to dress up fish for a quick, family-friendly weeknight meal. Incorporating oats into the topping adds a boost of nutritious whole grains. If you can't find tilapia, you can substitute any white fish, or even salmon. Fish is an excellent source of healthy omega-3s, which fuel the development of your baby's brain and eyes.

⅓ cup rolled oats
¼ cup panko breadcrumbs
1 clove garlic, finely chopped
2 tablespoons parsley, finely chopped
½ teaspoon dried oregano
1 teaspoon lemon zest

¼ teaspoon salt
1½ tablespoons olive oil
4 tilapia fillets, about 6 ounces each
Lemon wedges, for serving
Salt and pepper, to taste

Preheat oven to 400°F.

Pulse the oats in a food processor or blender until finely ground. Mix the oats, breadcrumbs, garlic, parsley, oregano, lemon zest, ¼ teaspoon salt, and olive oil together in a bowl.

Place the tilapia fillets on a greased baking sheet or in an oven-safe skillet (cast-iron works well) and season them with a pinch of salt and pepper. Spoon the topping evenly on top. Bake in the oven for 10–12 minutes, or until fish is cooked through. Squeeze some lemon juice on top before serving.

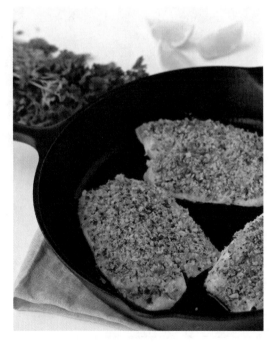

NUTRITIONAL INFORMATION

One serving: Calories 273; Fat 8.2g (Sat 1.9g); Protein 36.9g; Carbs 12g; Fiber 1.7g; Sodium 313mg

Veggie-licious Millet Cakes

Makes 12 cakes

Millet is a highly nutritious, gluten-free whole grain that forms the base of these crispy, savory cakes. Packed with nutritious vegetables, these fritters are an excellent addition to a vegetarian meal and also make a great finger food for baby.

1 cup low-sodium vegetable or chicken broth
½ cup millet
6 teaspoons olive oil, divided use
¼ cup finely chopped shallot or onion
1 carrot, peeled and grated

1 clove garlic, finely chopped
¼ teaspoon dried thyme
3 ounces (3 cups) baby spinach, chopped
¼ teaspoon salt
1 large egg and 1 egg white

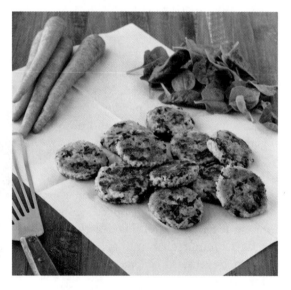

Bring the broth to a boil in a small saucepan and add the millet. Cover, reduce to a simmer and cook until soft, 15–20 minutes. Transfer the cooked millet to a large bowl.

Heat 2 teaspoons oil in a nonstick skillet over medium heat. Add the shallot, carrot, garlic, and thyme and cook for 2–3 minutes until partially softened. Add the spinach and cook until softened, another 2–3 minutes. Add the salt and stir to combine. Transfer the vegetables to the bowl with the cooked millet and cool. Add the eggs and stir to combine.

Form the mixture into 12 patties, about 2 tablespoons each, compacting them well. Heat 2 teaspoons oil in the skillet over medium heat. Add half of the patties to the pan and cook until golden brown, about 4–5 minutes. Flip and cook another 4–5 minutes on the second side. Remove from pan. Heat the remaining 2 teaspoons oil and cook the remaining patties.

Serve millet cakes with Greek yogurt or your favorite dipping sauce.

NUTRITIONAL INFORMATION

One cake: Calories 67; Fat 2.9g (Sat 0.5g); Protein 2.1g; Carbs 7.5g; Fiber 1.1g; Sodium 74mg

Sweet Potato and Kale Quesadillas

Makes 4 quesadillas

Kale is a leafy green vegetable that packs a nutritional punch! It contains powerful phytochemicals (natural, plant-based compounds) that are beneficial for your baby's health. It's also a rich source of several essential nutrients including Vitamin A, Vitamin C, Vitamin K, calcium and iron. Pairing kale with creamy sweet potatoes and black beans is a great way to introduce your little one to this superfood. Tuscan (lacinato) kale has a milder flavor than the more common curly variety. Serve these quesadillas with Greek yogurt or sour cream and your favorite salsa.

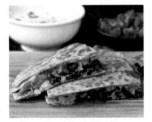

2 medium sweet potatoes, washed
¾ teaspoon chili powder
¼ teaspoon cumin
¼ teaspoon salt, divided use
3 teaspoons olive oil, divided use
1 clove garlic, finely chopped

3 cups chopped Tuscan or curly kale
4 large whole wheat tortillas
½ cup low sodium black beans, drained and rinsed
1 cup shredded cheddar cheese

Poke holes in the sweet potatoes with a fork. Roast them in the oven at 400°F until tender, 45-55 minutes. Alternatively, place them on a microwave-safe plate and cook in the microwave for 7–8 minutes until soft (turn them over halfway through). Let the potatoes cool then scoop out the flesh and place it in a bowl. Add the chili powder, cumin and 1/8 teaspoon salt and stir to combine.

Heat 1 teaspoon oil in a large cast iron or nonstick skillet over medium-high heat. Add the garlic and cook for 30 seconds until fragrant. Add the kale and 1/8 teaspoon salt and cook, stirring often, 4–5 minutes, until wilted. Remove kale from the skillet and place in a bowl. Wipe the skillet clean.

To assemble the quesadillas, place a tortilla on a flat surface and spread ¼ of the sweet potato mixture on one half of the tortilla. Spread ¼ of the kale on top of the sweet potato mixture and top with 2 tablespoons black beans and ¼ cup cheese. Fold the tortilla in half. Repeat with the remaining ingredients to make four quesadillas.

Heat 1 teaspoon oil in the skillet over medium heat and add two quesadillas. Cook 2–3 minutes until golden brown, then carefully flip the quesadillas and cook until golden brown on the second side. Remove from the pan and pour the remaining teaspoon oil in the skillet and cook the remaining two quesadillas.

Cut each quesadilla into four wedges and serve.

NUTRITIONAL INFORMATION

One quesadilla: Calories 372; Fat 13.6g (Sat 5.8g); Protein 14.7g; Carbs 50.7g; Fiber 7.7g; Sodium 653mg

Spinach & Artichoke Baked Potato Boats

Makes 4 servings

Who can resist cheesy potatoes? This twist on twice-baked potatoes incorporates nutritious vegetables—spinach and artichokes. Frozen artichoke hearts are a great time saver and are also economical. Feel free to incorporate your favorite ingredients in the filling like chopped broccoli, sundried tomatoes, or ham.

2 medium russet potatoes, scrubbed
1 teaspoon olive oil
1 clove garlic, finely chopped
2 ounces (2 cups) baby spinach, chopped
½ cup chopped artichoke hearts
1 tablespoon butter

3 tablespoons Greek yogurt or sour cream
½ cup plus 2 tablespoons shredded cheddar or Monterey Jack cheese, divided use
Salt and pepper, to taste

Preheat oven to 400°F.

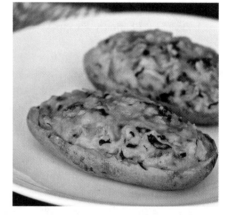

Pierce the potatoes in a few places with a fork and place them on a foil-lined baking sheet. Bake in the oven until cooked through, 50–60 minutes, turning over once during cooking. Remove from oven and cool.

While potatoes are baking, heat the oil in a skillet over medium heat. Add the garlic and cook until fragrant, about 30 seconds. Add the spinach and artichokes and cook 2–3 minutes, until spinach is wilted. Remove from heat.

Cut the potatoes in half lengthwise. Holding each potato with an oven mitt and using a spoon, carefully scoop out most of the filling into a bowl. Leave enough potato in the skin so that the shells stay together. Add the butter and yogurt to the potatoes and mash together with a fork until smooth. Stir in the spinach and artichoke mixture and ½ cup cheese. Taste, and season with a pinch of salt and pepper. Spoon the mixture back into the potato shells, mounding it slightly. Sprinkle the remaining 2 tablespoons cheese on top.

Place the potatoes on a baking sheet and bake in the oven until heated through, 15–20 minutes. Cool slightly and serve.

NUTRITIONAL INFORMATION

One serving: Calories 203; Fat 9.7g (Sat 5.9g); Protein 8.1g; Carbs 21.5g; Fiber 2.9g; Sodium 145mg

Baked Falafel

Makes about 18 falafel or 6 servings

Canned chickpeas are transformed into crispy, vegetarian fritters that are packed with protein, fiber, and flavor. Although falafel originated in the Middle East, it is popular all over the world. My version is baked instead of deep fried, making it much healthier.

2 cloves garlic
2 scallions
¼ cup fresh parsley
¼ cup fresh cilantro
2 cans (15.5 ounces each) low-sodium
    chickpeas, drained and rinsed
¼ cup flour
1 teaspoon ground cumin
1 teaspoon ground coriander
½ teaspoon baking powder
¾ teaspoon kosher salt
¼ teaspoon black pepper
1 tablespoon lemon juice
3 tablespoons olive oil

Tahini Yogurt Sauce
2 tablespoons tahini (sesame paste)
2 tablespoons plain Greek yogurt
1 tablespoon lemon juice
2–3 tablespoons warm water
Kosher salt, to taste

Preheat oven to 375°F.

Place the garlic, scallions, parsley, and cilantro in the bowl of a food processor and puree until finely chopped. Add the chickpeas, flour, cumin, coriander, baking powder, salt, pepper, and lemon juice. Pulse until the ingredients are incorporated and the chickpeas are ground, but not totally smooth.

Grease a baking sheet with 1½ tablespoons oil. Roll the chickpea mixture into 16 balls, approximately 1¼ inch each. Flatten each ball slightly to form thick patties and place them on the prepared pan. Brush the tops with the remaining 1½ tablespoons oil.

Bake in the upper third of the oven for 15 minutes, then flip and cook another 10–15 minutes until done. Meanwhile, make the tahini yogurt sauce by whisking the tahini, yogurt, lemon juice, and warm water together in a bowl. Taste, adding a pinch of salt if needed.

Serve the falafel with whole wheat pita, shredded Romaine lettuce, diced tomatoes and sliced cucumbers, if desired. Drizzle tahini yogurt sauce on top. Serve extra sauce on the side.

NUTRITIONAL INFORMATION

One serving (3 falafel plus sauce): Calories 251; Fat 11.6g (Sat 1.3g); Protein 9.1g; Carbs 29.1g; Fiber 6.9g; Sodium 495mg

Mac and Cheese with Roasted Cauliflower

Makes about 5 servings

Skip the boxed macaroni and cheese and make this dish instead! My mac and cheese is easy to make and so much healthier. It gets a nutritional boost from cauliflower, which is packed with powerful antioxidants as well as fiber, protein, and an impressive array of vitamins and minerals. Roasting the cauliflower in the oven caramelizes it and intensifies the flavor. You can substitute broccoli if you desire.

3 cups small cauliflower florets
1 tablespoon olive oil
8 ounces elbow macaroni, preferably whole grain
2 tablespoons unsalted butter
2 tablespoons flour
2 cups milk
½ teaspoon Dijon mustard
½ teaspoon salt
5 ounces shredded cheddar cheese (about 2 cups)
Salt and pepper, to taste

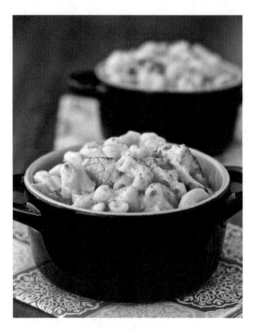

Preheat the oven to 425°F.

Place the cauliflower florets on a baking sheet lined with parchment paper. Toss the florets with the oil and a pinch of salt and pepper. Roast in the oven until edges are browned and cauliflower is cooked, 15–18 minutes.

Meanwhile, bring a large pot of water to a boil and cook the macaroni according to package directions. Drain.

Melt the butter in a large saucepan over medium heat. Add the flour and whisk until a smooth paste forms. Cook 1–2 minutes until the paste is light tan in color. Whisk in the milk, and bring to a simmer, whisking often, until a smooth sauce forms. Whisk in the mustard and ½ teaspoon salt. Simmer the sauce for a few minutes until it is thickened. Remove the pan from the heat and stir in the cheese until fully melted.

Add the cooked macaroni and roasted cauliflower to the sauce and stir to combine well.

NUTRITIONAL INFORMATION
One serving: Calories 425; Fat 19.8g (Sat 11.7g); Protein 18.5g; Carbs 44.4g; Fiber 5.1g; Sodium 479mg

Butternut Squash Tortellini Bake

Makes 6 servings

This comforting vegetarian baked pasta dish was shared by Matt Robinson over at Real Food by Dad (www.realfoodbydad.com). Matt is a fellow food blogger and loves to cook up delicious, family-friendly meals for his wife (also a talented food blogger) and three sons. Butternut squash is packed with nutrients and has a naturally rich, creamy texture that makes it perfect for incorporating into hearty sauces like this. The combination of sweet squash with earthy sage and sharp Parmesan cheese is out of this world! To cut down on prep time, you can purchase cubed, ready-to-cook squash from the grocery store.

1 pound peeled, cubed butternut squash	1 tablespoon flour
4 teaspoons olive oil, divided use	1½ cups milk
2 tablespoons unsalted butter	1 pound tortellini, cooked
6 sage leaves, thinly sliced	½ cup finely grated Parmesan cheese
½ cup chopped leeks	Salt and pepper, to taste

Topping
½ cup panko breadcrumbs, preferably whole wheat
2 tablespoons finely grated Parmesan cheese
1 tablespoon unsalted butter, melted

Preheat oven to 425°F.

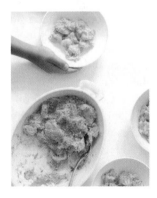

Place the squash on a baking sheet and drizzle with 2 teaspoons olive oil. Toss to coat, and sprinkle with a pinch of salt and pepper. Roast in the oven for 20–25 minutes or until slightly golden brown and fork tender. Remove from oven and set aside to cool. Transfer cooled butternut squash to a food processor or blender and blend until smooth. Set aside.

Melt the butter with the remaining 2 teaspoons olive oil in large skillet over medium-high heat. Add the sage leaves and cook for 1–2 minutes to infuse the oil with their flavor. Add the leeks and cook until soft and translucent, about 3 minutes. Sprinkle in the flour and whisk for 30 seconds.

Add the milk and pureed butternut squash and whisk to combine. Cook until thickened, 3–4 minutes. Stir in the Parmesan cheese. Taste, and season with a pinch of salt and pepper, if needed. Toss the sauce with the tortellini and transfer to a greased casserole pan.

To make the topping, combine the panko breadcrumbs and Parmesan cheese and toss with melted butter. Sprinkle evenly on top of the tortellini. Transfer the pan to the oven and broil for 2–3 minutes or until topping is golden brown. Cool slightly and serve.

NUTRITIONAL INFORMATION

One serving: Calories 449; Fat 17g (Sat 9.4g); Protein 17.8g; Carbs 54.6g; Fiber 4.1g; Sodium 660mg

Bacon and Egg Quinoa Fried Rice

Makes 4 servings

A healthier take on fried rice, my version of the dish features protein-packed quinoa and Canadian bacon. Canadian bacon is not a true cut of bacon but is rather a smoked cut of pork taken from the lean loin region. Cooled quinoa works best in this dish, so plan ahead and use leftover quinoa from the night before (or let it cool for a few hours in the fridge). This recipe is rich in protein, fiber, iron, and B vitamins.

1 cup quinoa, rinsed
4 teaspoons safflower, peanut, or other neutral-flavored oil, divided use
2 eggs
4 ounces Canadian bacon, diced
2 cloves garlic, minced
1 teaspoon minced ginger

1 cup frozen peas
2 tablespoons low-sodium soy sauce or tamari
2 teaspoons sesame oil
2 scallions, sliced (whites and greens separated)

Place the quinoa in a saucepan with 2 cups water and bring to a boil. Lower heat to a simmer and cover. Cook 10–15 minutes until done. Cool the quinoa, ideally overnight in the refrigerator.

Heat 1 teaspoon oil in a wok over medium high heat. Beat the eggs in a bowl with a fork and add them to the pan. Cook, stirring occasionally, until firm. Break the egg up into pieces with a spatula and transfer it to a plate.

Heat the remaining 3 teaspoons oil in the wok. Add the Canadian bacon and cook until lightly browned. Add the garlic, ginger, and scallion whites and cook until fragrant. Add the peas and cook 2-3 minutes until heated through. Add the cooled quinoa and stir to combine. Add the soy sauce, sesame oil, scallion greens, and cooked egg and stir to combine well.

NUTRITIONAL INFORMATION

One serving: Calories 320; Fat 12.5g (Sat 2.3g); Protein 16.3g; Carbs 34.4g; Fiber 4.8g; Sodium 629mg

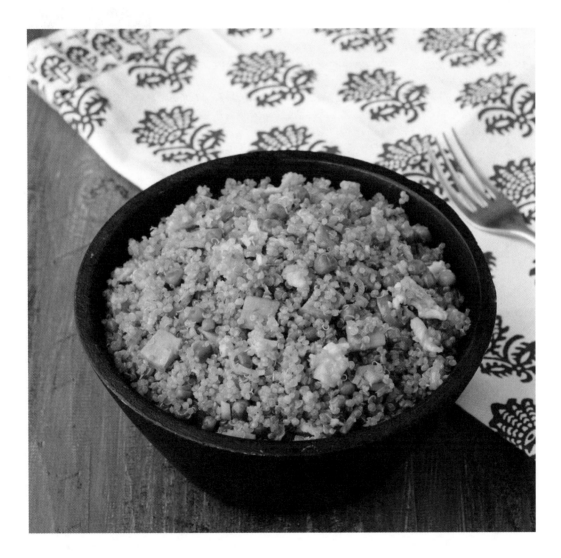

Spinach Gnudi

Makes 6 servings

Gnudi literally means "nude" in Italian, and that's exactly what they are—naked ravioli. Picture the filling in ravioli, minus the pasta: that's gnudi! Unlike gnocchi, which are primarily made with potatoes and flour, these light, pillow-like dumplings are made with ricotta cheese and egg and held together with just a small amount of flour. Spinach, nutmeg, and Parmesan cheese are also stirred into the mix for extra flavor. The result is a fluffy ball of goodness with a soft, creamy interior that both kids and adults will love.

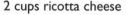

2 cups ricotta cheese
1 package (10 ounces) frozen chopped spinach, defrosted and squeezed very dry
4 large egg yolks
2.5 ounces (about ⅔ cup) grated Parmesan cheese (plus extra for garnish)

¼ teaspoon nutmeg
¾ teaspoon kosher salt
¼ teaspoon black pepper
1½ cups flour (all-purpose or white whole wheat), divided use
Veggie-Packed Tomato Sauce (page 229) or jarred lower-sodium marinara sauce, for serving

Mix the ricotta, spinach, egg yolks, Parmesan cheese, nutmeg, salt, and pepper together in a medium bowl until well combined. Stir in ½ cup flour until a sticky dough forms.

Pile the remaining cup of flour on a cutting board or plate. Drop a large spoonful of the dough (slightly larger than the size of a walnut) onto the flour and lightly toss it around in the flour until it is coated. Gently form the dough into a ball with your hands, shaking off any excess flour.

Repeat with the remaining dough. You should have about 24 gnudi in total. Discard the remaining flour. Meanwhile, bring a large pot of water to a boil, and then lower the heat to a simmer. Working in batches, gently lower the gnudi into the water. Cook the gnudi until they float to the surface of the water, about 4 minutes. Carefully remove them with a slotted spoon.

To serve, spoon some tomato sauce onto each plate and place the gnudi on top. Top with extra cheese, if desired.

NUTRITIONAL INFORMATION

One serving (4 gnudi): Calories 357; Fat 16.4g (Sat 10g); Protein 20.5g; Carbs 29.3g; Fiber 2.3g; Sodium 580mg

Cinnamon Roasted Sweet Potato Fries

Makes 4 servings

Making your own fries at home is so much healthier than buying them at a fast food restaurant, especially if you roast them in the oven and use sweet potatoes. Sweet potatoes have about the same amount of carbohydrates as white potatoes, but they're full of antioxidants, vitamins, minerals, and fiber. As your baby gets older, you can keep the skin on to retain more nutrients. Serve these fries with Turkey Sloppy Joes (page 235).

1 ½ pounds sweet potatoes (about 2 large potatoes), peeled and cut into batons (fry-shaped pieces)

2 tablespoons olive oil
½ teaspoon cinnamon
½ teaspoon kosher salt

Preheat oven to 425°F. Toss the sweet potatoes, oil, cinnamon, and salt together in a large bowl. Arrange them on a baking sheet in a single layer. Roast potatoes in the oven for 15 minutes, then flip them over and cook for another 8–10 minutes until cooked through. Serve warm.

NUTRITIONAL INFORMATION
One serving: Calories 206; Fat 6.6g (Sat 1g); Protein 2.7g; Carbs 34.5g; Fiber 5.3g; Sodium 384mg

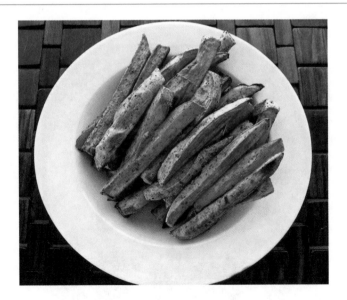

Miso Maple Roasted Carrots

Serves 4–6

Miso paste is a Japanese fermented soybean paste that can be found in Asian markets or specialty grocery stores. It comes in several different varieties, including white, yellow, and red. It adds rich, earthy flavor to this mildly sweet glaze that coats roasted carrots.

I pound carrots (about 6 medium carrots)
I tablespoon olive oil
I tablespoon white (shiro) miso paste

I tablespoon maple syrup
I teaspoon rice vinegar
I teaspoon low-sodium soy sauce

Preheat the oven to 400° F. Line a baking sheet with parchment paper and spray it with olive oil cooking spray. Peel the carrots and cut them on a bias into ⅓-inch slices.

Whisk the oil, miso paste, maple syrup, vinegar, and soy sauce together in a bowl. Add the carrots to the bowl and toss to coat them with the sauce. Transfer the carrots to the prepared baking sheet, spreading them out in a single layer.

Roast carrots in the oven until caramelized and tender, 20–25 minutes. Stir them once during cooking. Cool and serve.

NUTRITIONAL INFORMATION

One serving: Calories 98; Fat 3.7g (Sat 0.6g); Protein 1.6g; Carbs 15.5g; Fiber 3.4g; Sodium 282mg

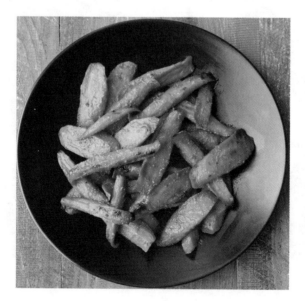

Green Beans and Sunshine

Makes 4 servings

Your little one will enjoy practicing their finger-feeding skills with these yummy green beans and oranges. Tossed in a simple dressing, this dish can be served warm or cold. It's a nice accompaniment to Salmon Cakes with Dilly Yogurt (page 244) or Barbecue Cheddar Mini Meatloaves (page 238).

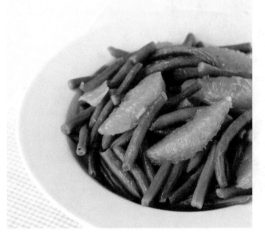

2 tablespoons olive oil
I tablespoon apple cider vinegar
½ teaspoon Dijon mustard
I teaspoon honey
I pound green beans, steamed
2 oranges, cut into segments*
Salt and pepper, to taste

Whisk the oil, vinegar, mustard, and honey together in a large bowl. Add the beans and oranges and toss to coat with the dressing. Season with a pinch of salt and pepper and serve.

NUTRITIONAL INFORMATION

One serving: Calories 132; Fat 6.9g (Sat 1g); Protein 2.7g; Carbs 17.1g; Fiber 4.6g; Sodium 94mg

> *To cut an orange into segments (also called supreming), first trim off the very top and bottom of the orange with a sharp knife. Then, set the orange on end and carefully cut the skin from the flesh, beginning at the top and following the curves down. Working over a bowl, cut in between the membranes to release the orange segments.

Apple Pie Quinoa
Cookies, page 264

Sweet
Treats

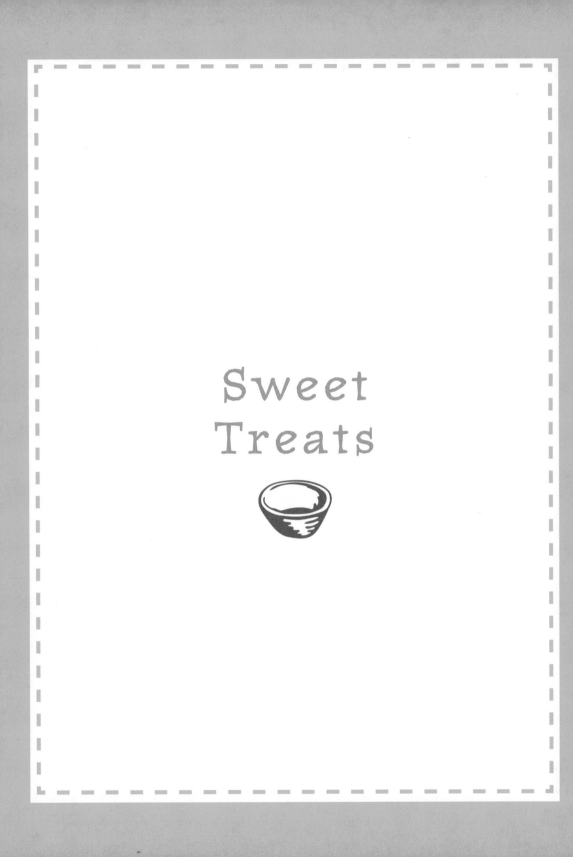

One-Ingredient Banana Ice Cream

Makes 4 servings

This one-ingredient ice cream is quick, easy, and nutritious—and you don't even need an ice cream maker! When you blend chopped up frozen bananas in a food processor, they are transformed into a deliciously rich and creamy dessert that tastes just like soft serve ice cream. It's a delicious, dairy-free treat that's rich in fiber as well as vitamin B6, vitamin C, potassium, and manganese. It also can be soothing for sore gums in teething tots.

4 ripe bananas, peeled

Cut the bananas into 1-inch pieces. Put them on a plate in a single layer and freeze until solid, at least 1–2 hours or overnight.

Place the frozen banana pieces in a food processor. Puree until creamy, about 2–3 minutes, scraping down the sides as needed. The ice cream can be served at this point, and will have a texture similar to soft serve ice cream. For a firmer texture, transfer the ice cream to an airtight container and place it in the freezer for at least an hour. Let the ice cream soften for about 10 minutes before serving.

Banana Peanut Butter variation: Add 2 tablespoons peanut butter to the ice cream and blend.

Banana Berry variation: Freeze 2 cups chopped strawberries with the bananas. Puree together in a food processor with ⅓ cup milk.

NUTRITIONAL INFORMATION

One serving: Calories 105; Fat 0.3g (Sat 0.1g); Protein 1.3g; Carbs 27g; Fiber 3.1g; Sodium 1mg

Super Strawberry Yogurt Pops

Makes 4 servings

Your little ones will love cooling off with this fun, three-ingredient recipe that comes straight from the wonderful blog, Meal Makeover Moms' Kitchen (www.mealmakeovermoms.com/kitchen). Made with fresh fruit and creamy yogurt, these all-natural pops are sweetened with 100 percent apple juice and have no added sugar. This recipe is flexible and can be adapted for all kinds of fruit so have fun experimenting with different combinations. Not only are these pops easy to make, but each one provides 12 percent of a toddler's daily requirement for calcium.

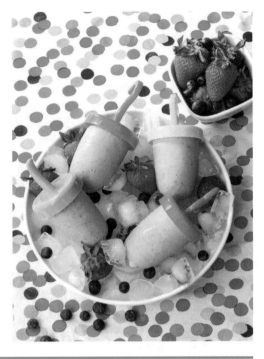

- 5 ounces (about 1 cup or 5–6 berries) fresh or frozen strawberries, stems removed and washed
- 1 cup strawberry yogurt
- ¼ cup 100 percent apple juice

Place the strawberries, yogurt, and juice in a blender and blend until smooth. Pour into four 3- or 4-ounce ice pop molds and freeze until firm, about 4 hours.

To remove the pops from the molds, run under warm water for about 20 seconds to loosen.

NUTRITIONAL INFORMATION

One pop: Calories 70; Fat 0.5g (Sat 0.3g); Protein 2g; Carbs 15g; Fiber 1g; Sodium 30mg

If you don't have ice pop molds, divide the liquid between four paper cups. Cover each cup with aluminum foil, insert one craft stick through the center of each piece of foil, and freeze.

Grilled Peaches with Greek Yogurt

Makes 4 servings

The next time you're having a barbecue, throw some fruit on the grill! Grilling fresh fruit caramelizes the natural sugars and deepens its flavor. If you don't have a grill, you can use a grill pan on your stove. Peaches are packed with vitamin C and also provide vitamin A, potassium, and fiber. Top them with a dollop of Greek yogurt for a boost of protein and calcium.

4 peaches, washed, halved, and pitted
2 teaspoons neutral-flavored oil like
    safflower or grapeseed
½ cup vanilla Greek yogurt
¼ teaspoon cinnamon
Optional toppings: drizzle of honey
    or raspberry puree, finely chopped
    almonds, or crushed graham crackers

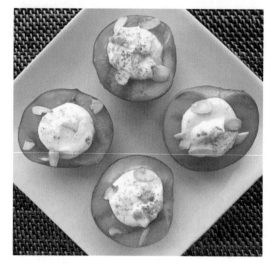

Heat a grill or grill pan over medium heat.

Brush the peaches with oil. Place them on the grill, cut side down, and cook until grill marks develop, 5–6 minutes. Flip the peaches over and cook another 3–4 minutes on the second side.

To serve, place a dollop of yogurt on each peach half and sprinkle cinnamon on top. If desired, add any additional toppings like a drizzle of honey or raspberry puree, finely chopped almonds, or crushed graham crackers.

NUTRITIONAL INFORMATION

One serving: Calories 104; Fat 2.8g (Sat 0.5g); Protein 2.9g; Carbs 18.7g; Fiber 2.3g; Sodium 20mg

Sri Lankan Fruit Salad with Whipped Vanilla Coconut Topping

Makes 8 servings

This refreshing fruit salad is packed with color, flavor, and essential nutrients. The recipe comes courtesy of my talented friend Shashi over at the site Runnin Srilankan (www.runninsrilankan. com). Shashi, a fellow mom and food blogger, takes a delightful blend of tropical fruits and pairs them with a creamy whipped vanilla coconut topping that takes this dessert to the next level!

1 ripe pineapple
1 ripe papaya
2 ripe mangoes
2 kiwi

2 bananas
1 vanilla pod
1 can full fat coconut milk (refrigerated)

Peel and chop the pineapple, papaya, mangoes, kiwi, and bananas and place them in a bowl. Let sit for about an hour so that all of the fruit juices can mingle.

Open the refrigerated can of coconut milk and scoop out the coconut cream (the semi-solid part that has risen to the top). Discard the water or reserve for another use. Place the coconut cream in a bowl. Scoop out the vanilla beans from the pod and place them in the same bowl. Using an electric mixer, whip the coconut cream and vanilla until well incorporated and fluffy.

Divide the fruit into bowls and top with dollops of the whipped vanilla coconut topping.

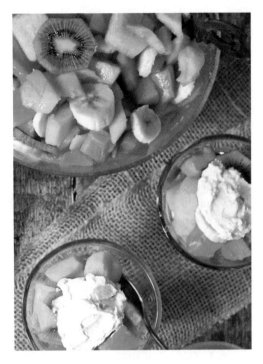

NUTRITIONAL INFORMATION

One serving: Calories 207; Fat 6.2g (Sat 5.5g); Protein 2.5g; Carbs 39.6g; Fiber 4.6g; Sodium 7mg

Coconut Whipped Cream

Made from coconut milk, this dairy-free whipped cream actually has no cream at all. All you need is a can of cold coconut milk. Refrigerate a can of full-fat coconut milk for several hours (light coconut milk won't work). Open the can and scoop out the solid coconut cream that has risen to the top (avoid shaking the can). You can save the remaining coconut water left in the bottom of the can for use in smoothies or other recipes. Place the coconut cream in a bowl and whip it with an electric mixer until it's fluffy like whipped cream. It will have a slightly sweet, coconut flavor.

Apple Pie Quinoa Cookies

Makes about 28 cookies

Kids and adults alike will enjoy these bite-sized treats, which are infused with the flavors of apple pie. Made with whole wheat flour, quinoa, and flaxseed, these nutritious cookies are packed with plenty of whole grains, protein, fiber, and omega-3s.

1½ cups white whole wheat flour
¼ cup ground flaxseed
½ teaspoon baking powder
½ teaspoon baking soda
1½ teaspoons cinnamon
½ teaspoon nutmeg
½ teaspoon kosher salt
1 cup cooked quinoa, cooled

½ cup melted coconut oil or unsalted butter
½ cup packed coconut sugar or light brown sugar
2 large eggs
1 teaspoon vanilla extract
1 large apple, peeled and grated (about ¾ cup)

Preheat oven to 350°F.

Line two baking sheets with parchment paper. Whisk the flour, flaxseed, baking powder, baking soda, cinnamon, nutmeg, and salt together in a large bowl. Add the quinoa and whisk to coat all of the grains with the flour mixture.

Using an electric mixer, beat the coconut oil and sugar together until well combined. Beat in the eggs and vanilla.

Add the flour mixture to the wet ingredients and mix until just combined (do not overmix). Squeeze all of the water out of the grated apple and add the apple to the mixer. Stir until just combined.

Spoon the dough in rounded tablespoons onto the prepared sheets, spacing them about 1 inch apart. Flatten them slightly with your hand (the cookies won't spread much during baking). Bake until golden, 15–18 minutes. Transfer cookies to a wire rack and let cool.

Note: Store cooled cookies in an airtight container at room temperature for up to two days, or freeze for up to one month.

NUTRITIONAL INFORMATION

One cookie: Calories 91; Fat 4.7g (Sat 3.6g); Protein 1.9g; Carbs 10.3g; Fiber 1.6g; Sodium 79mg

Sweet Potato Coconut Custard

Makes 4 servings

Nutrient-packed sweet potatoes are mixed with rich, creamy coconut milk and baked in the oven in this delicious dessert. The result is a silky-smooth custard that can be served warm or chilled. It will please both kids and adults and makes a lovely addition to your holiday table.

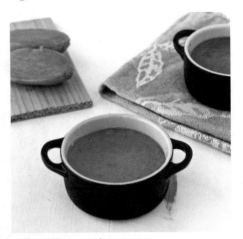

1 cup sweet potato puree
2 eggs
1 cup coconut milk
1½ tablespoons pure maple syrup
½ teaspoon vanilla extract
⅛ teaspoon cinnamon

Preheat oven to 325°F.

Place all of the ingredients in a blender and blend until smooth.

Pour the mixture into four greased ramekins (or 1 medium casserole dish) and place them in a water bath. To do this, set the ramekins in a baking dish and pour hot water into the baking dish until it comes half way up the sides of the ramekins (try not to get any water into the ramekins). Carefully place the dish in the oven and bake for 1 hour, until custard is set.

Remove from oven and cool slightly before serving. Top with a dollop of fresh whipped cream or Coconut Whipped Cream (see page 263), if desired.

NUTRITIONAL INFORMATION

One serving: Calories 208; Fat 13.3g (Sat 11.4g); Protein 4.9g; Carbs 17.3g; Fiber 1.7g; Sodium 57mg

---

Baking in a Water Bath

Some recipes, like this one, involve baking food in a "water bath." A water bath is a pan of water placed in the oven. A smaller dish containing the food is then placed in the pan of water until it is partially submerged. A water bath adds moisture to the oven and also provides a slower, more even heat source than the direct heat of the oven. This is useful when baking desserts like custards and cheesecakes because it helps them cook evenly and prevents them from curdling, cracking, or getting rubbery.

One-Ingredient Banana
Ice Cream, page 260

General Nutrition Information for Children and Families:

American Academy of Pediatrics: HealthyChildren.org
www.healthychildren.org

Academy of Nutrition and Dietetics
www.eatright.org

USDA MyPlate
www.choosemyplate.gov

USDA Dietary Guidelines for Americans
cnpp.usda.gov/DGAs2010-PolicyDocument.htm

Special Supplemental Nutrition Program for Women, Infants, and Children (WIC)
www.fns.usda.gov/wic/women-infants-and-children-wic

Allergies and Asthma:

American Academy of Allergy, Asthma, and Immunology
www.AAAAI.org

Food Allergy Research and Education (FARE)
www.foodallergy.org

Breast-feeding:

La Leche League International
www.llli.org

Food Safety:

Food Safety
www.cdc.gov/foodsafety

Fight Bac! Partnership for Food Safety Education
www.fightbac.org

First Aid/CPR

American Red Cross
www.redcross.org

Organic Food:

Environmental Working Group
www.ewg.org

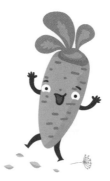

INDEX

A

ALA (alpha-linolenic acid), 32
Alaskan seafood, purity of, 48
allergies. *see* food allergies
almond butter
    Creamy Almond with Banana
        Wheels, 211
amino acids, 28
anaphylaxis, 40
anemia, 34, 47
Apple Pie Quinoa Cookies, 264
Apple Puree, 76
apples
    Apple Pie Quinoa Cookies, 264
    Apple Puree, 76
    Apple Strawberry Compote, 130
    banana ripening and, 187
    Gingery Carrots and Apples, 127
    Millet Porridge with Apples and
        Cinnamon, 150
    Purple Power (Blueberries, Kale,
        and Apple), 132
    Stewed Pork with Apple and
        Sweet Potato, 165
Apple Strawberry Compote, 130
Apricot Puree, 104
apricots
    Apricot Puree, 104
    Apricots, Bananas, and Barley,
        127
    Dried Plum (Prune) Puree
        (variation), 108–109
Apricots, Bananas, and Barley, 127
artichoke
    Spinach and Artichoke Baked
        Potato Boats, 248
asparagus
    Asparagus in a Blanket, 198–199
Asparagus in a Blanket, 198–199
Avocado Egg Salad, 204
Avocado Mash, 81
avocados
    Avocado Egg Salad, 204
    Avocado Mash, 81
    Avocado Yogurt Dip, 213

    Black Beans, Mango, and
        Avocado, 122
    Classic Avocado Toast, 210
    Salmon and Avocado Mash, 116
Avocado Yogurt Dip, 213

B

baby food containers, 53
Baby's Beef Puree, 114
Baby's Bolognese, 164–165
Baby's Burrito Bowl, 159
Baby's Chicken Curry, 163
Baby's Chicken Puree, 112–113
Baby's First Barley Cereal, 86
Baby's First Oatmeal Cereal, 87
Baby's First Pasta, 153
Baby's First Rice Cereal, 85
Baby's Fish Dinner, 116
background of book, vi
Bacon and Egg Quinoa Fried Rice,
    252
Baked Falafel, 249
baking ingredients, essential, 56
Banana Date Oat Muffins, 187
Banana Mash, 80
bananas
    Apricots, Bananas, and Barley,
        127
    Banana Berry Ice Cream
        (variation), 260
    Banana Date Oat Muffins, 187
    Banana Mash, 80
    Banana Peanut Butter Ice Cream
        (variation), 260
    Blueberry Banana Puree, 107
    Creamy Almond with Banana
        Wheels, 211
    One-Ingredient Banana Ice
        Cream, 260
    Peachy Banana Oatmeal, 150
    Peanut Butter Banana Smoothie,
        218
    Pumpkin Banana Delight, 126
    Pumpkin Banana Snack Bites,
        209

    ripening, 187
    Roasted Bananas and Pears,
        136–137
    Sri Lankan Fruit Salad with
        Whipped Vanilla Coconut
        Topping, 262–263
    Tropical Tofu Smoothie Bowl,
        169
Barbecue Cheddar Mini
    Meatloaves, 238
barley
    Apricots, Bananas, and Barley,
        127
    Baby's First Barley Cereal, 86
    Barley, 144
    Beef and Barley with Pumpkin,
        163–164
Barley, 144
Basic Brown Rice, 144
Basil, Strawberries, Beets, and, 167
beans. *see also specific types*
    foods to choose, 18
    solid foods, starting, 10, 13
Beautiful Beet Hummus, 216
beef
    Baby's Beef Puree, 114
    Baby's Bolognese, 164–165
    Barbecue Cheddar Mini
        Meatloaves, 238
    Beef and Barley with Pumpkin,
        163–164
    Sunday Beef Stew, 236
Beef and Barley with Pumpkin,
    163–164
Beet Puree, 99
beets
    Beautiful Beet Hummus, 216
    Beet Puree, 99
    solid foods, starting, 10
    Strawberries, Beets, and Basil,
        167
berries. *see also specific types*
    Banana Berry Ice Cream
        (variation), 260

Cherries, Berries, and Yogurt, 126

Very Berry Smoothie, 216–217

Black Bean Puree, 121

black beans

  Baby's Burrito Bowl, 159

  Black Bean Puree, 121

  Black Beans, Mango, and Avocado, 122

Black Beans, Mango, and Avocado, 122

blackberries

  Strawberry Puree (variation), 107

blender use, 13, 51–52, 139

blue baby syndrome, 47

blueberries

  Blueberry Banana Puree, 107

  Blueberry Dutch Baby, 189

  Blueberry Maple Compote, 190

  Blueberry Puree, 106

  Purple Power (Blueberries, Kale, and Apple), 132

  Whipped Ricotta with Blueberries, 168

Blueberry Banana Puree, 107

Blueberry Dutch Baby, 189

Blueberry Maple Compote, 190

Blueberry Puree, 106

boiling, avoidance of, 33, 50

Bolognese, Baby's, 164–165

bottle feeding. *see also* breast milk or formula

  phasing out, 13, 92, 180

  solid food caution, 9

botulism, 25

Bread, Cauliflower Cheesy, 202

breakfast

  Banana Date Oat Muffins, 187

  Blueberry Dutch Baby, 189

  Blueberry Maple Compote, 190

  Breakfast Burrito Bites, 191–192

  Cheesy Scrambled Eggs, 190–191

  Peaches and Cream Baked Oatmeal, 192

  Pumpkin Spice Quinoa Porridge, 194

  sample feeding schedule, 64

  sample menus, 93, 141, 181

  Southwest Breakfast Scramble (variation), 191

  Strawberry and Cream Cheese Stuffed French Toast, 195

  Sweet Potato Pancakes, 188

Breakfast Burrito Bites, 191–192

breast milk or formula

  cow's milk comparison, 24

  food allergies and, 40

  iron levels, 34

  macronutrients overview, 31

  micronutrients overview, 36

  nitrate contamination and, 47

  palate development and, 19

  sample feeding schedule, 64

  solid food, starting, 6–7, 9, 11, 13–14, 64

  vegetarian diets and, 37–38

broccoli

  Broccoli, Peas, and Pear, 129

  Broccoli Puree, 96–97

  Cheesy Quinoa Broccoli Bites, 175

  Chicken, Broccoli, and Rice Skillet Bake, 230

  Jolly Green Baked Potato, 152

  Roasted Broccoli Pesto, 212

Broccoli, Peas, and Pear, 129

Broccoli Puree, 96–97

Burrito Bowl, Baby's, 159

butternut squash

  Butternut Squash Puree, 69

  Butternut Squash Risotto, 128–129

  Butternut Squash Tortellini Bake, 251–252

  Cherries, Butternut Squash, and Millet, 157

  Lentils, Leeks, and Squash, 156

Butternut Squash Puree, 69

Butternut Squash Risotto, 128–129

Butternut Squash Tortellini Bake, 251–252

C

calcium

  foods to choose, 18, 24

  iron absorption and, 35

  micronutrients overview, 36

  sample food plan, 180

  vegetarian diets and, 37

canned foods

  essential foods, 57

  foods to choose, 45

cannellini beans

  Pasta Fagioli, 222

cantaloupe

  Cantaloupe, Peaches, and Cottage Cheese, 128

Melon Puree, 109

Cantaloupe, Peaches, and Cottage Cheese, 128

carbohydrates

  foods to choose, 18

  macronutrients overview, 29–31

  simple vs. complex, 29–30

Carrot Puree, 72

carrots

  Carrot Puree, 72

  Gingery Carrots and Apples, 127

  Miso Maple Roasted Carrots, 256

  Orange Crush (Carrots, Mango, and Nectarine), 133

  Pastina with Orange Sauce, 154

  Roasted Root Vegetable Trio, 136

  Salmon with Lentils and Carrots, 166–167

cauliflower

  Cauliflower Cheesy Bread, 202

  Cauliflower Puree, 97

  Cheesy Cauliflower Rice, 160

  Mac and Cheese with Roasted Cauliflower, 250

  Red Lentil and Cauliflower Puree, 121

Cauliflower Cheesy Bread, 202

Cauliflower Puree, 97

cereals. *see also* grains; *specific types*

  Baby's Beef Puree (variation), 114

  Baby's Chicken Puree (variation), 112–113

  Baby's First Barley Cereal, 86

  Baby's First Oatmeal Cereal, 87

  Baby's First Rice Cereal, 85

  essential foods, 56

  feeding caution, 9

  food preparation, 84

  foods to choose, 18

  micronutrients overview, 34

  solid foods, starting, 9, 10, 12–13

cheeses. *see also specific types*

  Barbecue Cheddar Mini Meatloaves, 238

  Cauliflower Cheesy Bread, 202

  Cheesy Cauliflower Rice, 160

  Cheesy Quinoa Broccoli Bites, 175

  Cheesy Scrambled Eggs, 190–191

  foods to avoid, 24, 25

foods to choose, 18, 26
Goldfish Crackers, 203
Grilled Cheese Dippers with Creamy Tomato Sauce, 173
Mac and Cheese with Roasted Cauliflower, 250
micronutrients overview, 35
solid foods, starting, 13
Sweet Potato Coins with Cheese, 176
Cheesy Cauliflower Rice, 160
Cheesy Quinoa Broccoli Bites, 175
Cheesy Scrambled Eggs, 190–191
cherries
   Cherries, Berries, and Yogurt, 126
   Cherries, Butternut Squash, and Millet, 157
   Cherry Puree, 103–104
Cherries, Berries, and Yogurt, 126
Cherries, Butternut Squash, and Millet, 157
Cherry Puree, 103–104
chicken
   Baby's Chicken Curry, 163
   Baby's Chicken Puree, 112–113
   Chicken and Rice Dinner, 161
   Chicken, Broccoli, and Rice Skillet Bake, 230
   Chicken Corn Chowder, 162
   Chicken, Mango, and Quinoa, 160
   Chicken Parmesan Sliders, 234
   Creamy Chicken and Corn Taquitos, 232
   dark vs. white meat, 113
   Pasta with Creamy Tomato Sauce and Chicken Sausage, 233
   Pretzel-Crusted Chicken Tenders with Honey Mustard Dipping Sauce, 226–227
Chicken and Rice Dinner, 161
Chicken, Broccoli, and Rice Skillet Bake, 230
Chicken Corn Chowder, 162
Chicken, Mango, and Quinoa, 160
Chicken Parmesan Sliders, 234
chickpeas
   Baked Falafel, 249
   Chickpeas, Spinach, and Pumpkin, 155
   Classic Hummus, 214

Chickpeas, Spinach, and Pumpkin, 155
chill food safety step, 55
choking
   activity caution, 181
   bottle feeding caution, 9
   choking/CPR guidelines, 43–44, 269–270
   finger foods caution, 172
   foods to avoid, 25, 43, 139–140
Chowder, Chicken Corn, 162
Cinnamon, Millet Porridge with Apples and, 150
Cinnamon Roasted Sweet Potato Fries, 255
Classic Avocado Toast, 210
Classic Hummus, 214
clean food safety step, 54–55
coconut milk
   Coconut Rice with Sweet Potatoes, 158
   Coconut Whipped Cream, 263
   Sri Lankan Fruit Salad with Whipped Vanilla Coconut Topping, 262–263
   Sweet Potato Coconut Custard, 265
   Tropical Rice Pudding, 131
Coconut Rice with Sweet Potatoes, 158
Coconut Whipped Cream, 263
combinations and combination meals
   Apple Strawberry Compote, 130
   Apricots, Bananas, and Barley, 127
   Baby's Bolognese, 164–165
   Baby's Burrito Bowl, 159
   Baby's Chicken Curry, 163
   Baby's First Pasta, 153
   Beef and Barley with Pumpkin, 163–164
   Broccoli, Peas, and Pear, 129
   Butternut Squash Puree, 69
   Cantaloupe, Peaches, and Cottage Cheese, 128
   Cheesy Cauliflower Rice, 160
   Cherries, Berries, and Yogurt, 126
   Chicken and Rice Dinner, 161
   Chicken Corn Chowder, 162
   Chicken, Mango, and Quinoa, 160

Chickpeas, Spinach, and Pumpkin, 155
Coconut Rice with Sweet Potatoes, 158
Creamy Split Pea Soup, 155
Fish with Mushy Peas, 166
Gingery Carrots and Apples, 127
Hawaiian Sweet Potato Casserole, 168–169
introduction, vi, 63, 90, 140
Jolly Green Baked Potato, 152
Lentils, Leeks, and Squash, 156
Millet Porridge with Apples and Cinnamon, 150
Orange Crush (Carrots, Mango, and Nectarine), 133
Pastina with Orange Sauce, 154
Peachy Banana Oatmeal, 150
Pumpkin Banana Delight, 126
Purple Power (Blueberries, Kale, and Apple), 132
Risi e Bisi, 158–159
Salmon with Lentils and Carrots, 166–167
solid foods, starting, 10, 12–13
Stewed Pork with Apple and Sweet Potato, 165
Strawberries, Beets, and Basil, 167
Tropical Rice Pudding, 131
Tropical Tofu Smoothie Bowl, 169
Whipped Ricotta with Blueberries, 168
Yellow Lentils and Rice (Khichdi), 129–130
compotes
   Apple Strawberry Compote, 130
   Blueberry Maple Compote, 190
constipation, 15, 30
contamination concerns. see food safety
cook food safety step, 55
Cookies, Apple Pie Quinoa, 264
cookie sheets, for freezing food, 53
cooking food preparation step, 49, 50–51
corn
   Chicken Corn Chowder, 162
   Creamy Chicken and Corn Taquitos, 232
Cottage Cheese, Cantaloupe, Peaches and, 128
cow's milk. see milk, cow's

CPR, choking/CPR guidelines, 43–44, 269–270
CPR classes, 43
Crackers, Goldfish, 203
cream cheese
  Pineapple Cream Cheese Spread, 174
  Strawberry and Cream Cheese Stuffed French Toast, 195
Creamy Almond with Banana Wheels, 211
Creamy Chicken and Corn Taquitos, 232
Creamy Pumpkin Dip, 213
Creamy Split Pea Soup, 155
Creamy Tomato Sauce and Chicken Sausage, Pasta with, 233
Crispy Tofu Nuggets, 200
cross-contamination, avoiding, 55
cup, drinking from, 13, 92, 140, 180
Curry, Baby's Chicken, 163
Custard, Sweet Potato Coconut, 265

D
dairy products. *see also specific foods*
  essential foods, 58
  finger foods, 172
  foods to avoid, 24, 26
  foods to choose, 18
  iron absorption and, 35
  sample food plan, 180
Date Oat Muffins, Banana, 187
desserts. *see* sweet treats
DHA (docosahexaenoic acid), 18, 32, 48
diarrhea, 26, 30
diet and nutrition
  foods to avoid, v, 13, 16, 24–26, 41, 43, 47–48
  foods to choose, v, 16–24, 26, 45–48, 56–58
  homemade food benefits, v–vi, 3–5
  introduction, v–vi
  macronutrients overview, 28–32
  micronutrients overview, 32–36
  nutrition building blocks, 27–38
  resources, 267–268
  solid foods, starting, 6–15
  vegetarian diet, 36–38

Dilly Yogurt, Salmon Cakes with, 244
dinner
  Bacon and Egg Quinoa Fried Rice, 252
  Baked Falafel, 249
  Barbecue Cheddar Mini Meatloaves, 238
  Butternut Squash Tortellini Bake, 251–252
  Chicken, Broccoli, and Rice Skillet Bake, 230
  Chicken Parmesan Sliders, 234
  Cinnamon Roasted Sweet Potato Fries, 255
  Creamy Chicken and Corn Taquitos, 232
  Green Beans and Sunshine, 257
  Lamb Kofta Kebabs with Tzatziki Sauce, 240
  Mac and Cheese with Roasted Cauliflower, 250
  Miso Maple Roasted Carrots, 256
  Pasta with Creamy Tomato Sauce and Chicken Sausage, 233
  Pork and Vegetable Stir-Fry, 242
  Pretzel-Crusted Chicken Tenders with Honey Mustard Dipping Sauce, 226–227
  Salmon Cakes with Dilly Yogurt, 244
  sample feeding schedule, 64
  sample menus, 93, 141, 181
  Spinach and Artichoke Baked Potato Boats, 248
  Spinach Gnudi, 254
  Sunday Beef Stew, 236
  Sweet Potato and Kale Quesadillas, 247
  Tilapia Oreganata, 245
  Turkey Florentine Meatballs, 228
  Turkey Sloppy Joes, 235
  Veggie-licious Millet Cakes, 246
  Veggie-Packed Tomato Sauce, 229
Dippers, Grilled Cheese, with Creamy Tomato Sauce, 173
dips
  Avocado Yogurt Dip, 213
  Creamy Pumpkin Dip, 213

Dried Plum (Prune) Puree, 108–109
Dutch Baby, Blueberry, 189

E
Easy Soba Noodles, 206–207
eggs
  Avocado Egg Salad, 204
  Bacon and Egg Quinoa Fried Rice, 252
  Breakfast Burrito Bites, 191–192
  Cheesy Quinoa Broccoli Bites, 175
  Cheesy Scrambled Eggs, 190–191
  foods to avoid, 25
  foods to choose, 18, 48
  food temperature guide, 55
  solid foods, starting, 13
  Southwest Breakfast Scramble (variation), 191
  Spinach and Ham Mini Frittatas, 173–174
eight to twelve months old
  amount and frequency of feeding, 140–141
  choking/CPR guidelines, 269
  combinations, 150–169
  finger foods, 172–177
  grains, 144–146
  recipes introduction, 139–141
  sample menu, 141
  solid foods, starting, 11, 13–14
EPA (eicosapentaenoic acid), 18, 32
equipment, kitchen, 12, 49, 51–52
extrusion reflex, 6–7

F
Falafel, Baked, 249
fats, macronutrients overview, 31–32
feeding schedule, sample, 64
fertilizers, 46–47
fiber, macronutrients overview, 30
finger foods
  Cheesy Quinoa Broccoli Bites, 175
  Grilled Cheese Dippers with Creamy Tomato Sauce, 173
  introduction, 139–140, 172
  no-recipe foods, 172
  pincer grip and, 13, 139

Pineapple Cream Cheese Spread, 174
Sienna's Veggie Nuggets, 175–176
Spinach and Ham Mini Frittatas, 173–174
Sweet Potato Coins with Cheese, 176
Zucchini Fries, 177
first aid for choking. *see* choking
fish. *see also* seafood
  Fish with Mushy Peas, 166
  food safety, 55
  foods to avoid, 25
  foods to choose, 48
  Tilapia Oreganata, 245
fish purees
  Baby's Fish Dinner, 116
  Salmon and Avocado Mash, 116
  Super Salmon Puree, 115
Fish with Mushy Peas, 166
flaxseeds, about, 217
Florentine Meatballs, Turkey, 228
flour, white whole wheat, 204
folate, 18
food allergies
  foods to avoid, 24, 41
  nutrition building blocks, 39–42
  solid foods, starting, 10–11
food challenge tests, 42
food elimination trials, 42
food intolerance, 40–42
food labels
  for frozen foods, 53
  "sell by" dates, 56
  on whole grain packages, 30
food mill use, 52
food plan, sample, 180. *see also* menus, sample
food preparation
  cereals and grains, 84
  cooking step, 49, 50–51
  homemade food benefits, 4–5
  involving children, vi, 17
  kitchen equipment, 49
  preparation step, 49, 50
  pureeing step, 49, 51–52
  reheating, 54
  serving step, 49, 52
  storing step, 49, 53
  water-soluble vitamins and, 33, 50
food processor use, 13, 52, 139

food safety
  allergies and intolerance, 39–42
  chill step, 55
  choking prevention, 43–44
  clean step, 54–55
  cook step, 55
  mercury, 18, 48
  nitrates, 47–48
  reheating, 54
  separate step, 55
  solid food caution, 9
  temperature guide, 55
foods to avoid
  allergic reaction triggers, 41
  choking hazards, 25, 43
  cow's milk, 24
  honey, 25
  introduction, v, 16
  juice, 26
  low-fat foods, 26
  nitrates, 47–48
  raw milk cheeses, 25
  raw or undercooked meat, seafood, or eggs, 25
  salt, 25
  solid foods, starting, 13
  sugar, 25
foods to choose
  fresh vs. frozen, 45
  fruits and vegetables, 45–47
  healthy foods, 18
  herbs and spices, 19–23
  introduction, v, 16–17
  meat and eggs, 48
  organic vs. conventional, 46–47
  pantry essentials, 56–58
  seafood, 48–49
food thermometers, 55
formula. *see* breast milk or formula
four to six months old
  food safety, 39–40
  micronutrients overview, 34
  solid foods, starting, 6, 12
freezing guidelines, 53–56
French Toast, Strawberry and Cream Cheese Stuffed, 195
fresh vs. frozen foods, 45
Fried Rice, Bacon and Egg Quinoa, 252
Fries, Cinnamon Roasted Sweet Potato, 255
Fries, Zucchini, 177
Fritattas, Spinach and Ham Mini, 173–174

frozen foods
  essential foods, 58
  foods to choose, 45
fruit juice
  foods to avoid, 26
  introducing, 13, 140
fruit purees. *see also* combinations and combination meals
  Apple Puree, 76
  Apricot Puree, 104
  Baby's Beef Puree (variation), 114
  Baby's Chicken Puree (variation), 112–113
  Banana Mash, 80
  Blueberry Banana Puree, 107
  Blueberry Puree, 106
  Cherry Puree, 103–104
  Chicken and Rice Dinner (variation), 161
  Dried Plum (Prune) Puree, 108–109
  homemade food benefits, 4
  introduction, 91
  Mango Puree, 105–106
  Melon Puree, 109
  Papaya Puree, 105
  Peach Puree, 102
  Pear Puree, 77
  Plum Puree, 103
  Pretty in Pink Raspberry Pear Puree, 108
  solid foods, starting, 10–12
  Strawberry Puree, 107
  as sweetener, 24, 25
fruits. *see also specific types*
  essential foods, 58
  finger foods, 172
  food safety, 54–55
  foods to choose, 18, 45–47
  sample food plan, 180
Fruit Salad, Sri Lankan, with Whipped Vanilla Coconut Topping, 262–263

G

Gingery Carrots and Apples, 127
glucose, 29
Gnudi, Spinach, 254
Goldfish Crackers, 203
grains. *see also* cereals; *specific types*
  Baby's Beef Puree (variation), 114

Baby's Chicken Puree (variation), 112–113
Barley, 144
Basic Brown Rice, 144
essential foods, 56
finger foods, 172
food preparation, 84
foods to choose, 18
Millet, 145
Oatmeal, 145
Quinoa, 146
sample food plan, 180
Green Bean Puree, 96
green beans
Green Bean Puree, 96
Green Beans and Sunshine, 257
Green Beans and Sunshine, 257
Grilled Cheese Dippers with Creamy Tomato Sauce, 173
Grilled Peaches with Greek Yogurt, 261–262

H
ham
Spinach and Ham Mini Frittatas, 173–174
Hawaiian Sweet Potato Casserole, 168–169
health resources, 267–268
heme iron form, 25
hemoglobin levels, 34
herbs
foods to choose, vi, 19–23
homemade food benefits, 4
pantry essentials, 58
solid foods, starting, 13
homemade food benefits
economical and convenient, 4–5
fun, 5
introduction, v–vi
nutritious ingredients, 4
palate development, v, 3–4
taste and variety, 4
honey
foods to avoid, 25
Pretzel-Crusted Chicken Tenders with Honey Mustard Dipping Sauce, 226–227
Ricotta, Strawberries, and Honey, 211
solid foods, starting, 14
honeydew melon
Melon Puree, 109

Honey Mustard Dipping Sauce, Pretzel-Crusted Chicken Tenders with, 226–227
hummus
Beautiful Beet Hummus, 216
Classic Hummus, 214
Turkey and Hummus Pinwheels, 206
hydrogenation process, 31–32
hygiene, food. *see* food safety

I
ice cream and pops
Banana Berry Ice Cream (variation), 260
Banana Peanut Butter Ice Cream (variation), 260
One-Ingredient Banana Ice Cream, 260
Super Strawberry Yogurt Pops, 260–261
ice cube tray use, 53
ice pop molds, paper cups for, 261
immersion blender use, 52, 139
infants, choking/CPR guidelines, 269
iron
absorption tips, 35
cereals and, 84
cow's milk and, 24
foods to choose, 18
micronutrients overview, 34–35
sample food plan, 180
solid foods, starting, 6, 10, 12

J
Jolly Green Baked Potato, 152
juice. *see* fruit juice

K
kale
Purple Power (Blueberries, Kale, and Apple), 132
Sweet Potato and Kale Quesadillas, 247
Kebabs, Lamb Kofta, with Tzatziki Sauce, 240
Khichdi (Yellow Lentils and Rice), 129–130
kitchen supplies
equipment, 12, 49, 51–52
pantry essentials, 56–58

kiwis
Sri Lankan Fruit Salad with Whipped Vanilla Coconut Topping, 262–263
Tropical Tofu Smoothie Bowl, 169
Kofta Kebabs, Lamb, with Tzatziki Sauce, 240

L
lactose, digestion, 24, 42
lamb
Baby's Beef Puree (variation), 114
Lamb Kofta Kebabs with Tzatziki Sauce, 240
Lamb Kofta Kebabs with Tzatziki Sauce, 240
leeks
Lentils, Leeks, and Squash, 156
legume purees. *see also* combinations and combination meals
Black Bean Puree, 121
Lentil Puree, 120
Red Lentil and Cauliflower Puree, 121
solid foods, starting, 10, 13
legumes. *see also specific types*
essential foods, 58
finger foods, 172
foods to choose, 18
Lentil Puree, 120
lentils
Lentil Puree, 120
Lentils, Leeks, and Squash, 156
Red Lentil and Cauliflower Puree, 121
Salmon with Lentils and Carrots, 166–167
Yellow Lentils and Rice (Khichdi), 129–130
Lentils, Leeks, and Squash, 156
low-fat foods
foods to avoid, 26
foods to choose, 18
lunch and snacks
Asparagus in a Blanket, 198–199
Avocado Egg Salad, 204
Avocado Yogurt Dip, 213
Beautiful Beet Hummus, 216
Cauliflower Cheesy Bread, 202
Classic Avocado Toast, 210
Classic Hummus, 214

Creamy Almond with Banana Wheels, 211
Creamy Pumpkin Dip, 213
Crispy Tofu Nuggets, 200
Easy Soba Noodles, 206–207
Goldfish Crackers, 203
introduction, 140, 179
Peanut Butter Banana Smoothie, 218
Pita Pizzas, 208
Pumpkin Banana Snack Bites, 209
Ricotta, Strawberries, and Honey, 211
Roasted Broccoli Pesto, 212
sample feeding schedule, 64
sample menus, 93, 141, 181
solid foods, starting, 14
Tropical Green Smoothie, 217
Turkey and Hummus Pinwheels, 206
Very Berry Smoothie, 216–217
Zucchini Tots, 198

M
Mac and Cheese with Roasted Cauliflower, 250
macronutrients overview. *see also specific types*
carbohydrates, 29–31
fats, 31–32
macronutrients defined, 27
proteins, 28–29
Mango Puree, 105–106
mangos
Black Beans, Mango, and Avocado, 122
Chicken, Mango, and Quinoa, 160
Mango Puree, 105–106
Orange Crush (Carrots, Mango, and Nectarine), 133
Sri Lankan Fruit Salad with Whipped Vanilla Coconut Topping, 262–263
Tropical Rice Pudding, 131
Tropical Tofu Smoothie Bowl, 169
masher use, 12–13, 52, 139
mashes
Avocado Mash, 81
Banana Mash, 80
Salmon and Avocado Mash, 116

meal planning. *see* food plan, sample; menus, sample
meat. *see also specific types*
essential foods, 58
finger foods, 172
food safety, 54–55
foods to avoid, 25
foods to choose, 18, 48
solid foods, starting, 13
Meatballs, Turkey Florentine, 228
Meatloaves, Barbecue Cheddar Mini, 238
meat purees
Baby's Beef Puree, 114
Baby's Chicken Puree, 112–113
solid foods, starting, 10, 12
Turkey and Taters, 113
Melon Puree, 109
menus, sample, 93, 141, 181
mercury in seafood, 18, 48
methemoglobinemia, 47
micronutrients overview. *see also specific types*
calcium, 36
iron, 34–38
micronutrients defined, 27
vitamins, 32–33
microwave, thawing foods in, 54
milk, cow's
food safety, 40
foods to avoid, 24
foods to choose, 18
micronutrients overview, 35
sample food plan, 180
solid foods, starting, 13–14
millet
Cherries, Butternut Squash, and Millet, 157
Millet, 145
Millet Porridge with Apples and Cinnamon, 150
Veggie-licious Millet Cakes, 246
Millet, 145
Millet Porridge with Apples and Cinnamon, 150
minerals overview. *see* micronutrients overview
Miso Maple Roasted Carrots, 256
molar development, 13, 139
monounsaturated fats, 31
Muffins, Banana Date Oat, 187
Mushy Peas, Fish with, 166

N
nectarines
Orange Crush (Carrots, Mango, and Nectarine), 133
Peach Puree (variation), 102
Stone Fruit Medley, 137
nitrates, 47–48
no-cook purees
Apricot Puree, 104
Avocado Mash, 81
Banana Mash, 80
Blueberry Puree, 106
Cherry Puree, 103–104
Mango Puree, 105–106
Papaya Puree, 105
Peach Puree, 102
Plum Puree, 103
Strawberry Puree (variation), 107
non-heme iron form, 25
Noodles, Easy Soba, 206–207
nuggets
Crispy Tofu Nuggets, 200
Sienna's Veggie Nuggets, 175–176
nut butters, serving of, 25. *see also specific types*
nutrition. *see* diet and nutrition
nuts, essential foods, 58

O
Oatmeal, 145
oats and oatmeal
Baby's First Oatmeal Cereal, 87
Banana Date Oat Muffins, 187
Oatmeal, 145
Peaches and Cream Baked Oatmeal, 192
Peachy Banana Oatmeal, 150
quick cooking oats, making, 187
oils, essential, 58
omega-3 fatty acids, 18, 37–38, 48
One-Ingredient Banana Ice Cream, 260
open cup, introducing, 140, 180
Orange Crush (Carrots, Mango, and Nectarine), 133
oranges
Green Beans and Sunshine, 257
Orange Sauce, Pastina with, 154
Oreganata, Tilapia, 245
organic vs. conventional foods, 46–47

P

palate development
  foods to choose, 19
  homemade food benefits, v, 3–4
pancakes
  Blueberry Dutch Baby, 189
  Sweet Potato Pancakes, 188
pantry, essential foods, 56–58
Papaya Puree, 105
papayas
  Papaya Puree, 105
  Sri Lankan Fruit Salad with
    Whipped Vanilla Coconut
    Topping, 262–263
Parmesan Sliders, Chicken, 234
Parsnip Pear Soup, 223
parsnips
  Parsnip Pear Soup, 223
  Roasted Root Vegetable Trio,
    136
partially hydrogenated fats, 32
pasta
  Baby's Bolognese, 164–165
  Baby's First Pasta, 153
  Butternut Squash Tortellini
    Bake, 251–252
  Mac and Cheese with Roasted
    Cauliflower, 250
  Pasta Fagioli, 222
  Pasta with Creamy Tomato
    Sauce and Chicken Sausage,
    233
  Pastina with Orange Sauce, 154
Pasta Fagioli, 222
Pasta with Creamy Tomato Sauce
  and Chicken Sausage, 233
pasteurized products, 18, 25
pastina
  Baby's First Pasta, 153
  Pastina with Orange Sauce, 154
Pastina with Orange Sauce, 154
peaches
  Cantaloupe, Peaches, and
    Cottage Cheese, 128
  Grilled Peaches with Greek
    Yogurt, 261–262
  Peaches and Cream Baked
    Oatmeal, 192
  Peach Puree, 102
  Peachy Banana Oatmeal, 150
  Stone Fruit Medley, 137
Peaches and Cream Baked
  Oatmeal, 192
Peach Puree, 102

Peachy Banana Oatmeal, 150
peanut butter
  Banana Peanut Butter Ice Cream
    (variation), 260
  Peanut Butter Banana Smoothie,
    218
Peanut Butter Banana Smoothie,
  218
Pear Puree, 77
pears
  Broccoli, Peas, and Pear, 129
  Parsnip Pear Soup, 223
  Pear Puree, 77
  Pretty in Pink Raspberry Pear
    Puree, 108
  Roasted Bananas and Pears,
    136–137
peas
  Broccoli, Peas, and Pear, 129
  Creamy Split Pea Soup, 155
  Fish with Mushy Peas, 166
  Risi e Bisi, 158–159
  Sweet Pea Puree, 70
pesticide residues, 46
Pesto, Roasted Broccoli, 212
phosphorus absorption, 37
phytonutrients, 18
pincer grip, 13, 139
pineapple
  Hawaiian Sweet Potato
    Casserole, 168–169
  Pineapple Cream Cheese
    Spread, 174
  Sri Lankan Fruit Salad with
    Whipped Vanilla Coconut
    Topping, 262–263
  Tropical Green Smoothie, 217
Pineapple Cream Cheese Spread,
  174
Pita Pizzas, 208
Pizzas, Pita, 208
Plum Puree, 103
plums
  Dried Plum (Prune) Puree,
    108–109
  Plum Puree, 103
  Stone Fruit Medley, 137
poaching technique, 51
polyunsaturated fats, 31
Pops, Super Strawberry Yogurt,
  260–261
pork
  Pork and Vegetable Stir-Fry,
    242

Stewed Pork with Apple and
    Sweet Potato, 165
Pork and Vegetable Stir-Fry, 242
Porridge, Pumpkin Spice Quinoa,
  194
potatoes, sweet
  Chicken Corn Chowder, 162
  Cinnamon Roasted Sweet Potato
    Fries, 255
  Coconut Rice with Sweet
    Potatoes, 158
  Hawaiian Sweet Potato
    Casserole, 168–169
  mashed, 188
  Roasted Root Vegetable Trio,
    136
  Spinach and Sweet Potatoes,
    98
  Stewed Pork with Apple and
    Sweet Potato, 165
  Sweet Potato and Kale
    Quesadillas, 247
  Sweet Potato Coconut Custard,
    265
  Sweet Potato Coins with Cheese,
    176
  Sweet Potato Pancakes, 188
  Sweet Potato Puree, 68
  Turkey and Taters, 113
potatoes, white
  Baby's Fish Dinner, 116
  Jolly Green Baked Potato, 152
  Potato Puree, 73
  Spinach and Artichoke Baked
    Potato Boats, 248
  Turkey and Taters, 113
potato masher use, 12–13, 52, 139
Potato Puree, 73
poultry. *see also specific types*
  essential foods, 58
  food safety, 54–55
  foods to avoid, 25
  foods to choose, 18, 48
preparation step, 49, 50. *see also*
  food preparation
Pretty in Pink Raspberry Pear
  Puree, 108
Pretzel-Crusted Chicken Tenders
  with Honey Mustard Dipping
  Sauce, 226–227
proteins
  cow's milk and, 24
  foods to choose, 18, 24
  macronutrients overview, 28–29

sample food plan, 180
vegetarian diets and, 37
prunes
Dried Plum (Prune) Puree,
108–109
Pudding, Tropical Rice, 131
pumpkin
Beef and Barley with Pumpkin,
163–164
Chickpeas, Spinach, and
Pumpkin, 155
Creamy Pumpkin Dip, 213
foods to choose, 45
Pumpkin Banana Delight, 126
Pumpkin Banana Snack Bites,
209
Pumpkin Spice Quinoa Porridge,
194
Pumpkin Banana Delight, 126
Pumpkin Banana Snack Bites, 209
Pumpkin Spice Quinoa Porridge,
194
pureeing step, 49, 51–52
purees. *see also specific types*
homemade food benefits, 4
introduction, vi, 63, 91
solid foods, starting, 10, 12–15
Purple Power (Blueberries, Kale,
and Apple), 132

Q
Quesadillas, Sweet Potato and
Kale, 247
quick cooking oats, making, 187
quinoa
Apple Pie Quinoa Cookies, 264
Bacon and Egg Quinoa Fried
Rice, 252
Cheesy Quinoa Broccoli Bites,
175
Chicken, Mango, and Quinoa,
160
Pumpkin Spice Quinoa Porridge,
194
Quinoa, 146
Quinoa, 146

R
raspberries
Pretty in Pink Raspberry Pear
Puree, 108
Strawberry Puree (variation),
107

ravioli, "naked," 254
raw or undercooked foods
food safety, 54–55
foods to avoid, 25
Red Lentil and Cauliflower Puree,
121
refrigeration guidelines, 53–56
reheating, rules for, 54
rice
Baby's Burrito Bowl, 159
Baby's First Rice Cereal, 85
Bacon and Egg Quinoa Fried
Rice, 252
Basic Brown Rice, 144
Butternut Squash Risotto, 128–
129
Cheesy Cauliflower Rice, 160
Chicken and Rice Dinner, 161
Chicken, Broccoli, and Rice
Skillet Bake, 230
Coconut Rice with Sweet
Potatoes, 158
Risi e Bisi, 158–159
Tropical Rice Pudding, 131
Yellow Lentils and Rice
(Khichdi), 129–130
Rice Cereal, Baby's First, 85
ricer use, 52
rickets, 37
ricotta
Ricotta, Strawberries, and
Honey, 211
Spinach Gnudi, 254
Whipped Ricotta with
Blueberries, 168
Ricotta, Strawberries, and Honey,
211
Risi e Bisi, 158–159
Risotto, Butternut Squash,
128–129
Roasted Bananas and Pears,
136–137
Roasted Broccoli Pesto, 212
roasted recipes
Cinnamon Roasted Sweet Potato
Fries, 255
Miso Maple Roasted Carrots,
256
Roasted Bananas and Pears,
136–137
Roasted Broccoli Pesto, 212
Roasted Root Vegetable Trio,
136
Stone Fruit Medley, 137

Roasted Root Vegetable Trio, 136
roasting technique, 50

S
salmon
Salmon and Avocado Mash, 116
Salmon Cakes with Dilly Yogurt,
244
Salmon with Lentils and
Carrots, 166–167
Super Salmon Puree, 115
Salmon and Avocado Mash, 116
Salmon Cakes with Dilly Yogurt,
244
Salmon with Lentils and Carrots,
166–167
salt
foods to avoid, 25
solid foods, starting, 14
saturated fats, 31
sauces
essential foods, 58
Grilled Cheese Dippers with
Creamy Tomato Sauce, 173
Lamb Kofta Kebabs with
Tzatziki Sauce, 240
Pasta with Creamy Tomato
Sauce and Chicken Sausage,
233
Pastina with Orange Sauce, 154
Pretzel-Crusted Chicken
Tenders with Honey Mustard
Dipping Sauce, 226–227
Salmon Cakes with Dilly Yogurt,
244
Tahini Yogurt Sauce, for Baked
Falafel, 249
Veggie-Packed Tomato Sauce,
229
Sausage, Chicken, Pasta with
Creamy Tomato Sauce and, 233
seafood. *see also* fish; *specific types*
food safety, 54–55
foods to avoid, 25
foods to choose, 18, 48
seasonings, essential, 58. *see also*
herbs; spices
seeds, essential foods, 58
self-feeding, 13–14, 139, 179
"sell by" dates, 56
separate food safety step, 55
serving step, 49, 52
shellfish. *see* seafood
Sienna's Veggie Nuggets, 175–176

sippy cup, introducing, 13, 92
six months old
amount and frequency of
feeding, 63–64
cereals, 84–87
choking/CPR guidelines, 269
combinations, 90–93
fruit purees, 76–77
micronutrients overview, 34
nitrate guidelines, 47
no-cook purees, 80–81
recipes introduction, 63–64
sample feeding schedule, 64
solid foods, starting, 6, 10, 12–13
vegetable purees, 68–73
six to eight months old
amount and frequency of
feeding, 91–92
choking/CPR guidelines, 269
combinations, 126–133
fruits, 102–109
juices, starting, 26
legumes, 120–122
meat and fish, 112–116
recipes introduction, 91–93
roasted recipes, 136–137
sample menu, 93
solid foods, starting, 12–13
vegetables, 96–99
sleep, solid foods and, 8
Sliders, Chicken Parmesan, 234
Sloppy Joes, Turkey, 235
smoothies
about, 218
Peanut Butter Banana Smoothie,
218
Tropical Green Smoothie, 217
Tropical Tofu Smoothie Bowl,
169
Very Berry Smoothie, 216–217
snacks. see lunch and snacks
Soba Noodles, Easy, 206–207
sodium, foods to avoid, 25
solid foods, starting
amount and frequency of
feeding, 10, 11, 63–64, 91–92
bottle feeding caution, 9
breast milk or formula and, 6–7,
9, 11
full baby signs, 9
how to start, 8–9, 63, 91
introduction, v–vi
micronutrients overview, 34
order of introduction, 10–11

sample feeding schedule, 63–64
sleep and, 8
stages, 12–15
stool changes, 15
3-5 day rule, 10
when to start, 6–7
soups
Chicken Corn Chowder, 162
Creamy Split Pea Soup, 155
Gingery Carrots and Apples
(variation), 127
Parsnip Pear Soup, 223
Pasta Fagioli, 222
Southwest Breakfast Scramble
(variation), 191
soy products, essential foods, 58
spices
foods to choose, vi, 19–23
homemade food benefits, 4
pantry essentials, 57
solid foods, starting, 13
spinach
Chickpeas, Spinach, and
Pumpkin, 155
Spinach and Artichoke Baked
Potato Boats, 248
Spinach and Ham Mini
Frittatas, 173–174
Spinach and Sweet Potatoes, 98
Spinach Gnudi, 254
Spinach Puree, 98
Tropical Green Smoothie, 217
Turkey Florentine Meatballs,
228
Spinach and Artichoke Baked
Potato Boats, 248
Spinach and Ham Mini Frittatas,
173–174
Spinach and Sweet Potatoes, 98
Spinach Gnudi, 254
Spinach Puree, 98
Split Pea Soup, Creamy, 155
spoons, selecting, 9, 139
Spread, Pineapple Cream Cheese,
174
squash
Butternut Squash Puree, 69
Butternut Squash Risotto, 128–
129
Butternut Squash Tortellini
Bake, 251–252
Cherries, Butternut Squash, and
Millet, 157
Lentils, Leeks, and Squash, 156

Zucchini Puree, 72–73
Sri Lankan Fruit Salad with
Whipped Vanilla Coconut
Topping, 262–263
steaming technique, 50, 91
Stewed Pork with Apple and
Sweet Potato, 165
stewing technique, 51
Stew, Sunday Beef, 236
sticky foods, choking caution, 25,
43, 172
Stir-Fry, Pork and Vegetable, 242
Stone Fruit Medley, 137
stool, changes in, 15, 26, 30
storing step, 49, 53
strainer use, 52
strawberries
Apple Strawberry Compote, 130
Ricotta, Strawberries, and
Honey, 211
Strawberries, Beets, and Basil,
167
Strawberry and Cream Cheese
Stuffed French Toast, 195
Strawberry Puree, 107
Super Strawberry Yogurt Pops,
260–261
Strawberries, Beets, and Basil, 167
Strawberry and Cream Cheese
Stuffed French Toast, 195
Strawberry Puree, 107
straw use, introducing, 140
sugar lactose. see lactose
sugars
carbohydrates overview, 29
foods to avoid, 25, 26
Sunday Beef Stew, 236
sun exposure, Vitamin D and, 37
Super Salmon Puree, 115
Super Strawberry Yogurt Pops,
260–261
sweeteners, fruit purees as, 24, 25
Sweet Pea Puree, 70
Sweet Potato and Kale
Quesadillas, 247
Sweet Potato Coconut Custard,
265
Sweet Potato Coins with Cheese,
176
sweet potatoes. see potatoes, sweet
Sweet Potato Pancakes, 188
Sweet Potato Puree, 68
sweet tooth development claim,
11

sweet treats
  Apple Pie Quinoa Cookies, 264
  Grilled Peaches with Greek
    Yogurt, 261–262
  One-Ingredient Banana Ice
    Cream, 260
  Sri Lankan Fruit Salad with
    Whipped Vanilla Coconut
    Topping, 262–263
  Super Strawberry Yogurt Pops,
    260–261
  Sweet Potato Coconut Custard,
    265

T
tahini
  about, 214
  Tahini Yogurt Sauce, for Baked
    Falafel, 249
Tahini Yogurt Sauce, for Baked
  Falafel, 249
Taquitos, Creamy Chicken and
  Corn, 232
teething
  cold foods and, 109
  finger foods and, 139, 172
  sleep and, 8
temperature of food, 25, 54, 55
texture of food
  food preparation, 50–52
  introduction, 139, 179
  stages of solids, 12–15
thawing guidelines, 54
thermometers, food, 55
three months old, nitrate
  guidelines, 47
three to five day rule
  food safety, 40
  solid foods, starting, 10, 63, 91
Tilapia Oreganata, 245
Toast, Classic Avocado, 210
Toast, French, Strawberry and
  Cream Cheese Stuffed, 195
tofu
  Crispy Tofu Nuggets, 200
  Tropical Tofu Smoothie Bowl,
    169
tomato sauce
  Grilled Cheese Dippers with
    Tomato Sauce, 173
  Pasta with Creamy Tomato
    Sauce and Chicken Sausage,
    233

Veggie-Packed Tomato Sauce,
  229
tongue thrust reflex, 6–7
Tortellini Bake, Butternut Squash,
  251–252
Tots, Zucchini, 198
trans-fats, 31–32
Tropical Green Smoothie, 217
Tropical Rice Pudding, 131
Tropical Tofu Smoothie Bowl, 169
turkey
  Baby's Chicken Puree (variation),
    112–113
  Turkey and Hummus Pinwheels,
    206
  Turkey and Taters, 113
  Turkey Florentine Meatballs,
    228
  Turkey Sloppy Joes, 235
Turkey and Hummus Pinwheels,
  206
Turkey and Taters, 113
Turkey Florentine Meatballs, 228
Turkey Sloppy Joes, 235
twelve months old and up
  amount and frequency of
    feeding, 179–180
  breakfast, 187–195
  choking/CPR guidelines, 270
  dinner, 226–257
  fats, starting, 31
  food safety, 39–40
  foods to avoid, 24–26
  juices, starting, 26
  lunch and snacks, 198–218
  micronutrients overview, 34–36
  recipes introduction, 179–182
  sample food plan, 180
  sample menu, 181
  solid foods, starting, 14
  soups, 222–223
  sweet treats, 260–265
Tzatziki Sauce, Lamb Kofta
  Kebabs with, 240

U
unsaturated fats, 31–32

V
Vanilla Coconut Topping,
  Whipped, Sri Lankan Fruit
  Salad with, 262–263

vegan diets, 36–38. see also
  vegetarian diets
vegetable purees. see also
  combinations and combination
  meals
  Avocado Mash, 81
  Baby's Beef Puree (variation),
    114
  Baby's Chicken Puree (variation),
    112–113
  Baby's Fish Dinner, 116
  Beet Puree, 99
  Broccoli Puree, 96–97
  Butternut Squash Puree, 69
  Carrot Puree, 72
  Cauliflower Puree, 97
  Chicken and Rice Dinner
    (variation), 161
  Green Bean Puree, 96
  homemade food benefits, 4
  Potato Puree, 73
  solid foods, starting, 10–12
  Spinach and Sweet Potatoes, 98
  Spinach Puree, 98
  Sweet Pea Puree, 70
  Sweet Potato Puree, 68
  Turkey and Taters (variation),
    113
  Zucchini Puree, 72–73
vegetables. see also specific types
  essential foods, 58
  finger foods, 172
  food safety, 54–55
  foods to choose, 18, 45–47
  Pork and Vegetable Stir-Fry, 242
  sample food plan, 180
  Sienna's Veggie Nuggets, 175–
    176
  Veggie-licious Millet Cakes, 246
  Veggie-Packed Tomato Sauce,
    229
vegetarian diets, micronutrients
  overview, 35, 36–38
Veggie-licious Millet Cakes, 246
Veggie-Packed Tomato Sauce, 229
Very Berry Smoothie, 216–217
Vitamin A, micronutrients
  overview, 31, 32–33
Vitamin B complex, micronutrients
  overview, 32–33
Vitamin B12, vegetarian diets
  and, 37
Vitamin C, micronutrients
  overview, 32–33, 35

Vitamin D
micronutrients overview, 31,
32–33, 36
sample food plan, 180
vegetarian diets and, 37
Vitamin E, micronutrients
overview, 31, 32–33
Vitamin K, micronutrients
overview, 31, 32–33
vitamins, 33. *see also specific
vitamins*
boiling and, 33, 50
overview of, 32–33

W

washing, as food safety step, 50,
54–55
water bath, baking in, 265
well water contamination, 47
Whipped Cream, Coconut, 263
Whipped Ricotta with Blueberries,
168
Whipped Vanilla Coconut
Topping, Sri Lankan Fruit
Salad with, 262–263

whole foods, choosing, 16
whole grains. *see also specific types*
foods to choose, 18
macronutrients overview, 30
solid foods, starting, 10
Whole Grain Stamp, 30
whole wheat flour, white, 204

Y

Yellow Lentils and Rice (Khichdi),
129–130
yogurt
Avocado Yogurt Dip, 213
Cherries, Berries, and Yogurt,
126
Creamy Pumpkin Dip, 213
foods to avoid, 24
foods to choose, 18, 26
Grilled Peaches with Greek
Yogurt, 261–262
Lamb Kofta Kebabs with
Tzatziki Sauce, 240
micronutrients overview, 35
Peachy Banana Oatmeal
(variation), 150

Salmon Cakes with Dilly Yogurt,
244
solid foods, starting, 13
Super Strawberry Yogurt Pops,
260–261
Tahini Yogurt Sauce, for Baked
Falafel, 249

Z

zinc
foods to choose, 18
solid foods, starting, 10
vegetarian diets and, 37
zucchini
Zucchini Fries, 177
Zucchini Puree, 72–73
Zucchini Tots, 198
Zucchini Fries, 177
Zucchini Puree, 72–73
Zucchini Tots, 198